Ketosis Cookbook

109 Ketogenic Diet Recipes That Confuse Your Body into BURNING Body Fat as Energy

(Breakfast, Lunch, Dinner & Snacks Recipes Included)

by Sarah Talene

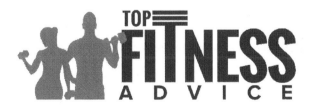

Sarah Talene
TopFitnessAdvice.com

Table of Contents

INTRODUCTION 4

HOW TO USE THIS BOOK 5

CHAPTER 1: BREAKFAST 7

CHAPTER 2: LUNCH 25

CHAPTER 3: DINNER 68

CHAPTER 4: SNACKS 119

CONCLUSION 127

FINAL WORDS 127

DISCLAIMER 129

Introduction

When it comes to commonly held beliefs, most people have been told that eating too much fat is what makes us sick. Whilst it is true that eating too many calories in a day is bound to lead to weight gain, cutting out fat is also not the answer. Fat came under fire because it is very calorie dense. It seems to make sense – cut out the more nutrient dense food in order to drop the number of calories that you consume.

However, if you consider that we evolved as hunter-gatherers who might have had to go without food for a day at a time or more, the picture becomes more complicated. Our bodies are not built for having such ready access to food in general and carbs in particular. Our ancestors had to go out and hunt for their food. Today though, we just stop in at the store. Pair that with our increasingly sedentary lifestyles and it is hardly surprising that we are becoming more obese and that dieting is such a huge trend. But, despite the fact that the typical low-fat diet has been punted as the best option for the last few decades, we are getting more obese. Despite us cutting out so much fat, we are increasingly unable to lose the weight. But look for a minute at what it is that we do eat. We take the fat out of food and it no longer tastes so good so we add in tons of sugar. The typical Western diet consists of a high level of processed foods that are high in sugar.

However, these highly processed carbs have very little nutrient value and, because they are so processed, they have a massive impact on our blood sugar levels. We eat the carbs and our blood sugar levels skyrocket. The body responds by increasing the production of insulin. The sugar is mopped up and your energy levels plummet again. You then crave even more carbs to fuel your body. You quickly get caught in a vicious cycle – you need the carbs for energy but they cause your blood sugar levels to crash fairly quickly. And, after the crash, your body requires more energy and so you have to eat again. If this happens over and over again, your body becomes less responsive to the insulin produced by it. You end up needing more insulin to clear out the excess blood sugar. More insulin is produced but it is less effective than before.

More of the glucose that is produced is left over in the blood stream and is converted to fat that gets stored in the body. The way to get out of this cycle, is to fuel your body in a completely different way. That is where a ketogenic diet comes in to play. Ketosis can reverse this by forcing your body to use the fat stores for energy. The ketogenic diet turns our commonly held belief about weight-loss on its head. Instead of cutting out as much fat as possible, you eat a diet that is high in protein and that has moderate amounts of fat and that restricts carbs as much as possible.

With the lack of glucose as a fuel source in the diet, the body has no choice but to start burning through the fat stored in it. Your body actually changes its preferred fuel source over to fat – and that is why you need to increase the amount of fat that you eat. The benefits of a ketogenic diet is that you will not feel hungry or deprived in any way and you will be able to lose weight easily. Once the initial adjustment period is over, you will find that you have a lot more energy and a greater ability to focus. We are not going to go into the actual diet in full in this book but we do provide you with recipes that are all keto-friendly. Good luck!

How to Use This Book

Choose one breakfast, one lunch, one dinner and either one or two snacks a day and you will start to feel the benefits for yourself. Unless otherwise stated, the following will apply to all recipes:

- All temperatures are in Fahrenheit.

- Do no use foods that are sweetened already – if necessary, the recipe will list what sweetener to use.

- Use organic, naturally produced food wherever possible.

Read This FIRST - 100% FREE BONUS

FOR A LIMITED TIME ONLY – Get Sarah's best-selling book *"The #1 Weight Loss Guide: The ONLY Book You Will Need to Read to Lose Weight FOREVER!"* absolutely FREE!

Readers who have read this bonus book as well have seen the greatest changes in their health and weight loss both *QUICKLY & EASILY* and have improved overall fitness levels – so it is *highly recommended* to get this bonus book.

Once again, as a big thank-you for downloading this book, I'd like to offer it to you *100% FREE for a LIMITED TIME ONLY!*

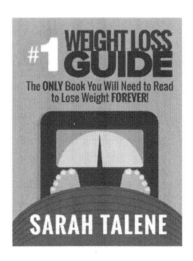

To download your FREE copy, go to:

TopFitnessAdvice.com/Freebie

Chapter 1: Breakfast

1. Chocolate Chia Cereal

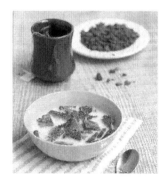

Serves 4

Ingredients

- 1 cup of plain
- ½ cup chia seeds
- 4 tablespoons hemp hearts
- 2 tablespoons melted coconut oil
- 1 tablespoon powdered psyllium
- 1 tablespoons vanilla extract essence
- 2 tablespoons cacao nibs, raw
- 1 tablespoon sweetener of your choice

Method

Set your oven at 285 and mix together the water and chia seeds and put them to one side for a few minutes so the seeds swell a little. Keep the nibs to one side and add all else to the bowl and mix together till a pliable dough is formed. Now you can add in the nibs. Lay down parchment paper, with the dull side facing down, to create a 11 x 14-inch sheet. Create a roll of dough that is around 13 inches long. Lay it onto the paper and begin to flatten out your dough. Take a second sheet of parchment paper and lay it over the dough. When that is in place, roll the dough until you get it to about a 1/8th of an inch thick.

Take out of the oven and take off the paper. Bake the dough for a further 25 minutes so that it dries out well. Let it cool off and then cut it up into squares of about an inch. Keep in a sealed container for three days at most.

2. Morning Coffee Porridge

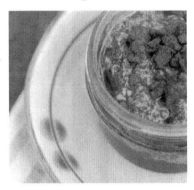

Serves 2

Ingredients

- ⅓ cup chia seeds
- 2 tablespoons coffee
- 2 tablespoons cacao nibs
- ⅓ cup coconut cream
- 1 tablespoons Sweetener of your choice
- 1 tablespoons vanilla extract essence

Method

Make a cup of strong coffee and then mix with the cream, sweetener and the extract. Then add in the nibs and the seeds. Mix well and refrigerate for no less than half an hour. The porridge is now ready. Use more coffee if you want a more liquid porridge.

3. Porridge from The Heart

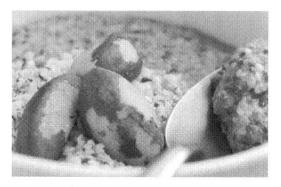

Serves 1

Ingredients

- ½ cup Hemp Hearts
- 1 cup non-dairy milk
- 2 tablespoons flax seed, ground
- 1 tablespoon sweetener of your choice
- 1 tablespoon chia seeds
- ¾ teaspoon vanilla extract essence
- ¼ cup crushed almonds
- ½ teaspoon powdered cinnamon, powdered

Ingredients for Toppings

- 1 tablespoon Hemp Hearts
- 3 Brazil nuts

Method

Blend the ingredients except for your chosen toppings and the crushed almonds and place in a small pot. Set your stove to Medium and bring the mix to a boil, stirring all the time. Simmer for a minute or two. Take off the heat and serve with the almonds and toppings.

4. Best "Cereal" In the Universe

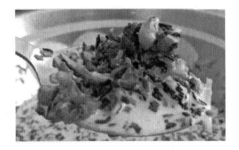

Serves 1

Ingredients

- 1/2 cup of grated coconut
- 4 teaspoons farm butter
- 2 cups non-dairy cream
- A touch of salt
- Sweetener, should you want it
- 1/3 cup of flaxseeds, lightly toasted
- 1/3 cup of either macadamia or walnut bits

Method

Set the stove to Medium and melt the farm butter. Put in the nuts and coconut and fry lightly until it starts to turn golden brown. Stir all the time so that nothing burns. Add the salt. Mix in the sweetener if you are using it and then stir the milk in fast. Remove from the stove and either serve immediately or set aside for a few minutes.

5. Egg "Porridge"

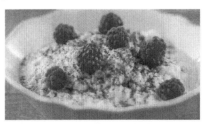

Serves 1

Ingredients

- 1/3 cup double cream
- 2 fresh eggs
- Powdered cinnamon
- 2 tablespoons farm butter
- Sweetener if you want it

Method

Mix together the cream, sweetener and eggs and mix properly. Set your stove to Med-High and heat the butter until just melted. Reduce the heat to low and add in the cream and egg. Stir gently and continuously and heat until the mixture starts to get thicker and curdles starts to form. When the first curdle forms, remove from the heat and serve with powdered cinnamon.

6. Cream Cheese Pancakes

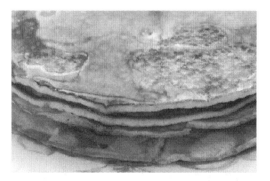

Makes 4 pancakes

Ingredients

- 2 eggs
- 2 ounces plain cream cheese
- ½ teaspoon powdered cinnamon

- 1 teaspoon granular sweetener

Method

Blend everything till completely smooth. Coat a non-stick pan with non-stick spray. Set your stove to Med-High and heat the pan. Pour around a fourth of the mixture into it and cook until bubbles start to appear on the surface. Flip the pancake and cook it for another minute or so. Do the same to make the other pancakes. Serve hot.

7. Almond Joy Pancakes

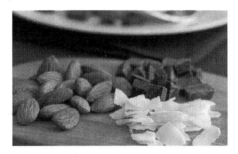

Serves 12

Ingredients

- 1/3 cup grated coconut
- 1/2 cup coconut flour
- 1/4 cup sweetener
- 1/2 teaspoon table salt
- 1/2 teaspoon baking powder
- 6 large eggs
- 1/2 - 1 cup plain non-dairy milk
- 1/4 cup coconut oil melted
- 1 teaspoon almond extract
- 2 ounces grated dark chocolate
- 1/4 cup slivered almonds, lightly toasted
- Oil for frying

Method

Mix together all the dry ingredients. Add the oil, the eggs, and half of the milk. You don't want batter that is quite as thin as pancake batter but it should be easy to spread in the pan. Should the batter thicken on standing you may need to add more milk. Add the nuts and chocolate. Set your stove to Med-High. Lightly oil a skillet and heat it up. Spoon around two large tablespoonfuls of the batter into your skillet and swirl so that it makes a circle of about 4 inches. Fit as many as you can into the skillet and cook until bubbles start to form and then flip. Cook until done.

8. Keto Pumpkin Pancakes

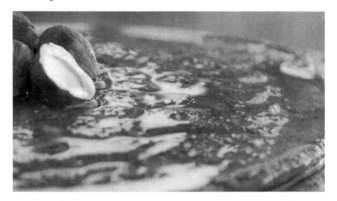

Serves 3

Ingredients

- 1 ounce egg white protein
- 2 ounces of hazelnuts, ground
- 1 teaspoon baking powder
- 1 teaspoon vanilla extract essence
- 1 tablespoon Chai Masala Mix
- 1 cup coconut cream
- ½ cup pumpkin puree
- 3 eggs
- 4 drops stevia glycerite

- Oil for frying
- Additional sweetener if you want it.

Method

Place all of the wet ingredients into a bowl and whisk well. In a separate bowl, mix together the flowers, seasoning, sweetener, stevia and baking powder. Add to the wet ingredients a little bit at a time, whisking well. You want a thicker batter that is still easy to pour. Set your stove to Med-High and coat a pan with some oil. Ladle the batter into the pan, turn the heat to low. Cover the pan and cook for a couple of minutes before flipping. Serve straight away.

9. French Toast

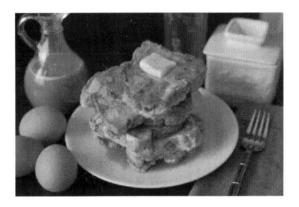

Serves 18

Ingredients for Bread

- 4 ounces plain cream cheese, at room temperature
- 1 cup whey protein
- 12 eggs, separated

Ingredients for French Toast

- ½ cup non-dairy milk
- 1 teaspoon powdered cinnamon

- 2 eggs
- 1 teaspoon vanilla extract essence

Ingredients for Syrup

- ½ cup Sweetener
- ½ cup farm butter
- ½ cup non-dairy milk

Method

Bread: Set your oven to 325. Whip the eggs whites until they form stiff peaks. Fold in the whey powder. Fold in the cream cheese. Grease your bread tins and divide the dough between them. Bake till golden brown (Around 40 minutes or so.) Don't cut until entirely cool. Freeze what you don't use.

French Toast: Set your stove to Med-High and grease a heavy-based frying pan. Mix together two of the eggs, the vanilla extract essence, the cinnamon and the milk. Dip your first slice of the bread into your mixture and put into the hot pan. Fry until nicely golden and flip. Do the same with the rest of the bread.

Syrup: Set your stove to High and put the butter into a heavy-based pot. Make sure that all the ingredients are ready and close because you need to act quickly. As soon as the butter starts to froth, add in your sweetener and then the milk. Whisk till it is a smooth sauce. Let it cool off and use. It will last for two weeks if refrigerated.

10. Waffle On

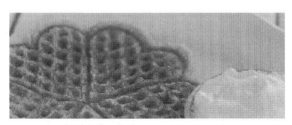

Servings 5

Ingredients

- 4 tablespoons coconut flour
- 5 eggs separated
- 3-5 tablespoons sweetener
- 1-2 teaspoon vanilla extract
- 1 teaspoon baking powder
- 4.5 ounces of melted farm butter
- 3 tablespoons fresh cream

Method

Whisk together the egg whites until stiff peaks form and set aside. In another bowl, mix the flour, egg yolks, baking powder and sweetener until completely combined. Add the butter bit by bit so that there are no lumps. Whisk in the vanilla extract and milk and then fold in the egg whites. Cook the waffles as you normally would.

11. Spicy Home-Made Granola

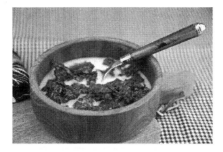

Serves 4

Ingredients

- 1/2 cup walnuts
- 1 cup pecans, coarsely chopped
- 1/2 cup almonds, coarsely chopped

16

- 1/2 cup almond flour
- 1/2 cup coconut flakes
- 1/4 cup chia seeds, finely ground
- 1/4 cup sunflower seeds
- 1/4 cup pumpkin seeds
- 1/4 cup melted farm butter
- 1 teaspoon honey
- 1/2 cup sweetener
- 1/4 cup of plain water
- 1 teaspoon vanilla extract
- 1 teaspoon powdered cinnamon
- 1/2 teaspoon salt
- 1/2 teaspoon nutmeg

Method

Set your oven to 250. Mix everything together well. Grease a baking tray and line it with baking paper. Spoon the granola on top as evenly as possible. Take another sheet of baking paper and place on top. Using a rolling pin, apply pressure and make sure that the granola is firmly packed and evenly spread. Throw out the covering sheet of baking paper and place in the oven. Let it cook for around an hour to an hour and a half or till it starts to turn golden. Let it cool and then break up into bite-sized bits.

12. Pumpkin Pie Granola

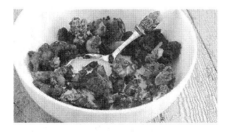

Serves 8

Ingredients

- ½ cup each of macadamia and pecan nuts, coarsely chopped
- 1 cup almonds, coarsely chopped
- 1 cup coconut flakes
- 1 cup desiccated coconut
- ½ cup pumpkin seeds
- ½ cup whey protein powder
- ¼ cup chia seeds
- ¼ cup sweetener
- ¼ teaspoon salt
- 1 tablespoon and 1 teaspoon pumpkin pie spice mix
- 10-15 drops liquid Stevia extract
- 1 large egg white
- ½ cup pumpkin puree
- ¼ cup melted coconut oil

Method

Set your oven to 300. Put the nuts into a bowl and mix. Add the coconut, the seeds, sweetener and the whey protein powder. Add the spices and salt. Mix in the oil, the stevia and the egg white and mix thoroughly. Add in the pumpkin. Spread the granola onto a tray nice and evenly. Bake it until it crisps up. (About half an hour). Set it aside to cool completely before serving. Store in an air-tight container for up to four weeks.

13. Granola for Health Nuts

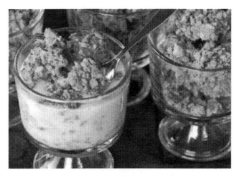

Serves 12

Ingredients

- 1/2 cup chopped walnuts
- 2 cups chopped pecans
- 1/2 cup slivered almonds
- 1 3/4 cup whey protein
- 1 cup sunflower seeds
- 1/2 cup sesame seeds
- 1/2 cup Sweetener
- 1 1/4 cup farm butter
- 1 teaspoon stevia glycerite
- 1/2 teaspoon salt
- 1 teaspoon powdered cinnamon

Method

Set your oven to 300 degrees F. Mix together everything except the butter. Melt the butter and then mix into the granola. Grease a baking tin and line with baking paper. Spoon the granola on evenly and bake it until it starts to turn golden. (About 20 minutes.) Cool completely and serve. Store leftovers in an air tight container.

14. Granola Without the Grains

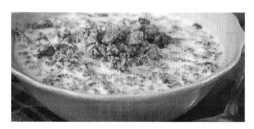

Serves 4

Ingredients

- 8 ounces of raw assorted nuts – without salt
- 1/3 cup erythritol
- 1/4 teaspoon table salt
- 1 extra large egg white
- 1/2 teaspoon powdered cinnamon

Method

Set your oven at 350. Grease a shallow baking tin and line with baking paper. Process the nuts until it is a meal. Mix in the rest of the ingredients and spread evenly over the baking tin. It should be a thin, even layer. Bake until it just starts changing color. (About 8 minutes or so). The mixture can catch easily so watch. Let it cool off completely and break into little pieces. Store in an airtight container.

15. Your Full Breakfast

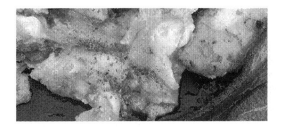

Serves 1

Ingredients

- 1 large peeled and sliced avocado
- 4 strips of sugar-free bacon
- ¼ teaspoon table salt
- 2 large eggs

20

Method

Set your stove to Medium and place the bacon and avocado in a non-stick pan. Fry for a few minutes on each side and put aside, keeping it warm. Fry your eggs in the bacon fat until done to your liking.

16. Zucchini Hash

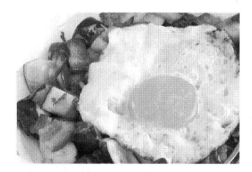

Serves 1

Ingredients

- 2 bacon rashers
- 1 medium zucchini
- ½ small onion
- ¼ teaspoon salt
- 1 tablespoon parsley, coarsely chopped
- 1 tablespoon coconut oil
- 1 large egg

Method

Chop the onion up nice and fine and cut the bacon into strips. Set your stove to Medium and fry your onion in a non-stick pan until soft. Add in your bacon and cook till a little brown. Set aside and cut up the zucchini. Fry in the same pan for about ten minutes or until done. Serve with the parsley.

17. Eggs and Sardines

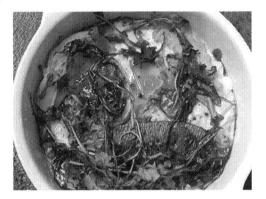

Serves 1

Ingredients

- 2 ounces of sardines packed in olive oil
- 2 eggs
- ½ cup arugula
- Seasoning to taste
- 2.5 tablespoons artichoke hearts

Method

Set your over to 375. Grease a small oven-proof dish and layer the sardines into it in one layer. Crack the eggs onto the sardines. Layer the artichokes and arugula. Season and bake for ten minutes or so.

18. Shakshuka

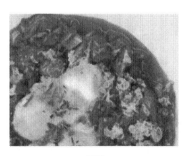

Serves 2

Ingredients

- 1 bell pepper
- 1 large onion
- 1.5 pounds cherry tomatoes
- ½ tablespoon cumin seeds
- ¼ cup extra virgin olive oil
- 2 thumb length thyme sprigs, picked off the stem
- Salt to taste
- Cayenne pepper to taste
- 1 tablespoon parsley, chopped up nice and finely
- 4 eggs

Method

Set your oven at 350. Halve the tomatoes. Grease a shallow baking tin and put the tomatoes onto it, cut side up, in a single layer. Season to taste. Bake until the tomatoes have started to caramelize and softened. (About half an hour.) Set your stove to Med-High and heat up a large frying pan. Dry fry the cumin until fragrant. Add in the oil and onions and change the heat to a Low setting. Fry until they soften. Cut the pepper into strips lengthwise and add to the pan. Add in the herbs and then the tomatoes. Season to taste. Bring the sauce to a boil, adding water if necessary. Crack the eggs over the mixture, keeping them separate from each other as far as possible. Set the stove to Low and cook for a further ten minutes or that the eggs are done to your liking.

19. Buttery, Herbed Eggs

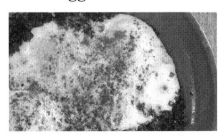

Serves 2

Ingredients

- 1 tablespoon coconut oil
- 2 tablespoons farm butter
- 2 garlic cloves, chopped up nice and fine
- ½ cup cilantro, chopped up nice and fine
- 1 teaspoon fresh thyme
- ½ cup freshly picked parsley, chopped up nice and fine
- ¼ teaspoon powdered cumin
- 4 eggs
- ½ teaspoon table salt
- ¼ teaspoon powdered cayenne

Method

Set your stove to Med-High and heat the oil and butter in a non-stick frying pan. Add in the garlic and reduce the temperature to Low. Cook until the garlic starts to turn brown. Stir in the thyme and fry for about a minute. Stir in the parsley and cilantro and fry until it starts to crisp up. Crack the eggs into the pan, cover it with a plate or a lid and fry for about five minutes or until the eggs are done to your liking. Serve while still warm.

20. Cheese Soufflé

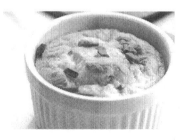

Serves 8

Ingredients

- 1 teaspoon salt
- 1/2 cup almond flour
- 1 teaspoon mustard powder
- 1/2 teaspoon xanthan gum
- Seasoning to taste
- 1/4 teaspoon cayenne pepper
- 2 cups mature cheddar cheese, grated
- 3/4 cup double cream
- 1/4 cup chives, chopped
- 1/4 teaspoon cream of tartar
- 6 large eggs, separated

Method

Set your oven at 350. Grease eight ramekins and place them on a large baking tray. Whisk the flour, xanthan gum and seasonings together until combined. Add the cream in until completely mixed. Add the egg yolks, chives and cheese and mix well. In a separate bowl, whisk the egg whites and the cream of tartar till it forms stiff peaks and looks glossy. Fold the egg whites into the other mixture until fully combined. Divide out the mixture evenly between all the ramekins and put in the oven. Bake until the soufflés have risen above the rim and start to go brown. Serve straight away.

Chapter 2: Lunch

1. Tasty Meat Pie

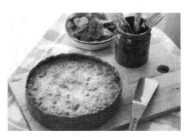

Serves 4-6

Ingredients for Filling

- 1 garlic clove, chopped up nice and finely
- 1 mild onion, chopped up nice and finely
- 2 tablespoons farm butter
- Seasoning to taste
- 1 1/3 pounds ground lamb or beef
- 1 tablespoon dried oregano
- ½ cup of plain water
- 4 tablespoons tomato paste

Ingredients for Pie Crust

- 4 tablespoons Sesame seeds
- ¾ cup almond flour
- 4 tablespoons coconut flour
- 1 teaspoon baking powder
- 1 tablespoon powdered psyllium husks
- 1 pinch salt
- 4 tablespoons water
- 1 egg
- 3 tablespoons olive or coconut oil

Ingredients for Topping

- 7 ounces of cheese, grated
- ½ pound cottage cheese

Method

Set your oven at 350.

Filling: Set your stove to Medium and melt the butter in a heavy-based pan. Fry the onion and garlic until they soften. Stir in the beef, minced and add in the seasoning and herbs. Stir well and fry until it starts to brown. Reduce the heat and allow the mixture to simmer for around 20 minutes, stirring every once in a while.

Pie Crust: Mix the ingredients for the dough together until they come together as a firm dough and are completely combined. Grease a baking tin or pie plate with a 10-inch diameter and line it with baking paper. Flatten the dough into the pie plate, ensuring that it covers both the bottom and the sides evenly. Bake it blind for ten minutes or so. Remove it from your oven and then spoon in the meat, again evenly. Mix together the topping ingredients and spoon over the top. Bake the pie for around half an hour or so – it should turn out to be a golden-brown color. Serve with a nice leafy salad.

2. Nested Eggs and Zucchini

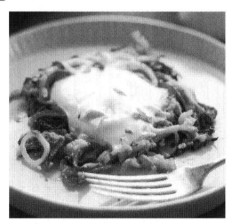

Serves 2

Ingredients

- 4 slices bacon
- 4 cups zucchini noodles
- ½ cup Cheddar, grated
- Seasoning to taste
- 4 eggs

Method

Cut the bacon into long, thin strips. Set your stove to High and fry the bacon until slightly crispy. Stir in the zucchini. Season to taste and create wells in the zucchini. Divide the cheese up between the wells and then crack the eggs into the wells. Set your stove to Med-High and cook for around 3 minutes. Cover the pan and continue to cook for another couple of minutes or until the eggs are cooked as you like them.

3. Deluxe Hamburgers

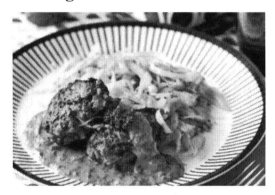

Makes 8

Ingredients for Hamburger Patties

- 1 egg
- 1½ pounds beef, minced
- 3¼ ounces of feta
- ¼ teaspoon powdered black pepper
- 1 teaspoon table salt
- 1¾ ounces of freshly picked parsley, chopped up nice and finely
- 1 ounces of farm butter
- 1 tablespoon olive oil

Ingredients for Gravy

- 1¾ ounces of freshly picked parsley, chopped up nice and finely
- 1¼ cups double cream
- 2 tablespoons tomato paste

Ingredients for Fried Cabbage

- Seasoning to taste
- 1½ pounds grated cabbage
- Seasoning to taste
- 4¼ ounces of farm butter

Method

Patties: Blend all the ingredients together and divide into eight equal sized balls. Flatten into patties. Set your stove to Med-High and met the farm butter and olive oil. Add the patties when hot and fry until they are almost done. Mix together the cream and tomato paste and pour into the pan. Bring the mixture to a boil. Set aside and keep warm while making the cabbage.

Fried Cabbage: Grate the cabbage. Set your stove to Medium and, in a clean pan, melt the butter. Fry up the cabbage until done, stirring occasionally – it should take about 15 minutes. Season to taste and serve with the burgers and sauce. Top with the parsley.

4. Stuffed Cabbage

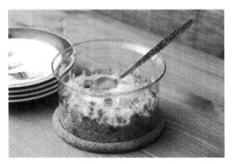

Serves 3-4

Ingredients

- 1/3 pound farm butter
- 1½ pounds cabbage, chopped up nice and finely
- 1 pound beef mince
- 1 teaspoon onion powder
- Salt and pepper to taste
- 2 tablespoons Tex-Mex seasoning
- 1 tablespoon white wine vinegar
- 1/3 pound leafy greens, like lettuce
- 2/3 pound Cheddar, grated

Method

Set your oven at 400. Set the stove to Med-High and melt the farm butter in a large wok. Cook until the cabbage softens but don't let it go brown. (Around about ten minutes or so.) Add in the vinegar and the spices. Fry for a few more minutes, stirring constantly. Put to the one side and keep warm. Using the same pan, fry up the beef, stirring continuously until it has browned. Reduce the heat to Med-Low. Stir in the cabbage and fry for a minute or two. Season as you like. Add in about two thirds of the cheese and transfer the mixture to a greased oven-proof dish. Top with the remaining cheese and put in the oven. Cook until the cheese starts to bubble and crisp up. It will take about 15 minutes.

5. Stir-Fried Cabbage

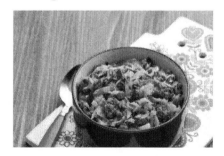

Serves 4

Ingredients

- 1/3 pound farm butter
- 1 2/3 pounds cabbage
- 1 1/3 pounds beef, minced
- 1 teaspoon onion powder
- Salt and pepper to taste
- 2 garlic cloves
- 1 tablespoon white wine vinegar
- 3 scallions, chopped into slices
- 1 tablespoon fresh ginger, chopped up nice and finely
- 1 teaspoon chili flakes
- 1 tablespoon sesame oil

Ingredients for Wasabi Mayo

- ½ – 1 tablespoon wasabi paste
- 1 cup mayo

Method

Grate the cabbage so that it is fine. Set your stove to Med-High. Add 2/3 of the farm butter and cook the cabbage in batches until softened but not brown. In in the vinegar and the rest of the spices and fry again. Set the cabbage aside in a bowl and keep warm. Add spices and vinegar. Stir and fry for a couple of minutes more. Put the cabbage in a bowl. Using the same pan, melt the leftover butter and add the ginger, chili and the garlic and cook for a couple of minutes until fragrant. Cook the meat throughout, ensuring that you stir regularly. Make sure just about all the pan juices are cooked out. Reduce the heat and stir in the cabbage and scallions. Make sure it is heated through. Add seasoning as required and finish off with sesame oil. Mix the wasabi and mayo together until you get the flavor that you are looking for. Serve with the food.

6. European Chicken Casserole

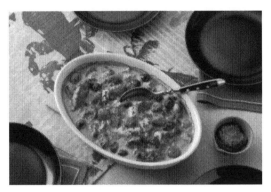

Serves 4-6

Ingredients

- 3 ½ ounces of pesto of your choice
- 1 ½ pounds chicken pieces – breasts or thighs, skinned and boned
- 1 2/3 cups double cream
- 1 garlic clove, chopped up nice and finely
- ½ pound feta cheese, chopped up into cubes
- 8 tablespoons olives, pits removed
- Farm butter, to fry the food in
- Seasoning to taste

Method

Set your oven at 400. Slice the chicken into bite-sized pieces. Season as you like. Set you stove to Med-High and melt the farm butter. Fry the chicken until done. Mix together the cream and the pesto. Grease an oven-proof dish and put the chicken pieces into it, in a single layer. Add the feta, the olives, garlic and the pesto. Put in oven and bake until heated through and bubbling hot. (About 25 minutes.)

7. Wrapped Dogs

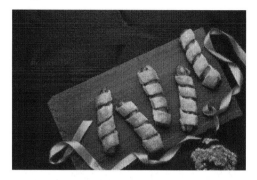

Makes 8

Ingredients

- 4 tablespoons coconut flour
- 8 tablespoons almond flour
- ½ teaspoon table salt
- 2 2/3 ounces of farm butter
- 1 teaspoon baking powder
- 1½ cups cheese, grated
- 8 long, good quality wieners
- 1 egg
- 1 egg, to brush onto the dough

Method

Set your oven at 350. Mix together the flours and the baking powder. Set your stove to Low and put the farm butter and cheese in a heavy-bottomed pan. Mix well, so that the batter is smooth and moldable. Take off the stove. Beat one of the eggs in a bowl and add the dry ingredients and cheese mixture so that the dough is firm. Roll out the dough so that it forms a large rectangle about 8 inches by 14 inches. Cut into eight equal strips. Grease a baking sheet and line it with baking paper. Wrap the wieners in the dough and then bake for about 15 minutes. The dough should be golden in color.

8. Low-Carb Pizza

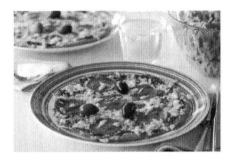

Serves 2

Ingredients for Crust

- 6¼ ounces of Provolone or Cheddar
- 4 eggs

Ingredients for Topping

- 1 teaspoon dried oregano
- 4 tablespoons tomato paste
- 4¼ ounces of cheese, grated
- Olives
- 1¾ ounces of Pepperoni

Method

Set your oven at 400. Beat together the eggs with the cheese. This will form the pizza base. Grease a baking sheet and line it with baking paper. Divide the dough into two equal parts. You can pour the batter onto the baking paper and spread the batter out in a circular shape. Bake for around 15 minutes or so until the crust is golden in color. Take out of the oven and let it cool off. Set your oven to 450. Divide the paste between the two crusts and add some oregano Put your olives, pepperoni and cheese on top. Put in the oven and bake until it is golden in color. Serve with a leafy salad.

9. Keto Hash Browns

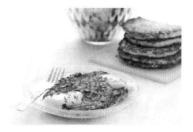

Serves 2

Ingredients

- 3 eggs
- 1 pound cauliflower
- ½ mild onion, grated
- 4 ounces of farm butter, to use to fry the food
- Seasoning to taste

Method

Clean the cauliflower and grate it up coarsely. Mix it and the rest of the ingredients together and allow them to marinate together for about 10 minutes or so. Set the stove to Medium and heat up the farm butter in a large frying pan. You want to be able to cook more than one hash-brown at a time. Drop the cauliflower mix into your frying pan one large spoonful at a time and press to flatten. Fry them for about 4 minutes and flip. Don't flip the hash-browns too early or they will crumble.

10. Creamy Chicken Casserole

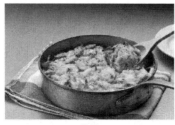

Serves 4

Ingredients

- 7 ounces of cheese, grated
- 2 pounds of chicken thighs
- 1¼ cups double or sour cream
- 1 leek
- 2/3 pound cauliflower, broken into florets
- 4 ounces of cherry tomatoes
- The juice of ½ lemon
- 2 tablespoons pesto
- 3 tablespoons farm butter
- Seasoning to taste

Method

Set your oven at 400. Mix together the pesto, lemon juice and the cream. Add seasoning as you like. Season the chicken and set the stove to Medium-High. Melt the farm butter in a large frying pan and cook the chicken until it turns golden and crispy. Grease an oven-proof baking dish. Put the chicken put in one layer and then add the cream. Slice up the leek nice and fine and halve the tomatoes. Put the tomatoes, cauliflower and leek over the chicken. Top with cheese and put in the oven. Cook for around about half an hour to forty-five minutes on the middle rack of your oven.

11. Spicy Mexican Casserole

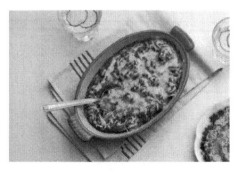

Serves 4

Ingredients

- 1½ pounds beef, minced
- 2 ounces of jalapeños
- 1 cup sour cream
- 7 ounces of cheese, grated
- 1 scallion, chopped up nice and finely
- Guacamole to taste
- 2 tablespoons farm butter
- 2 teaspoons chili powder
- 1 teaspoon powdered cumin
- 2 teaspoons paprika powder
- 1 – 2 teaspoons onion or garlic powder
- Salt as required
- Cayenne pepper to taste

Method

Set your oven at 400. Set your stove to Med-High. Melt the butter in a large frying pan. Put the mince in and add the tomatoes and seasoning. Grease an oven-proof dish and put the beef into it. Top with the cheese and chilis. Put on one of the uppermost racks in the oven and bake it for about 20 minutes or so. Serve topped with guacamole, cream and a leafy salad.

12. Keto Lasagna

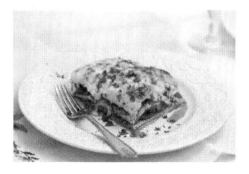

Serves 4

Ingredients

- 1 1/3 pounds beef, minced
- 2 tablespoons olive oil
- 1 mild onion
- 3 tablespoons tomato paste
- 1 garlic clove
- ½ tablespoon dried basil
- ½ cup of plain water
- Seasoning to taste

Ingredients for Keto Pasta

- 5 1/3 tablespoons powdered psyllium husks
- 2/3 pound cream cheese
- 8 eggs
- 1 teaspoon table salt

Ingredients for Cheese Topping

- 1/3 pound cheese, grated
- 2 cups sour cream
- 8 tablespoons freshly picked parsley, chopped up nice and finely
- 2 ounces of fresh Parmesan, grated
- Seasoning to taste

Method

If you have time, make the pasta sauce the day before and let the flavors develop overnight. To make the sauce, finely chop up the garlic and onion. Set your stove to Med-High and heat up the olive oil. Add in the garlic and onion and fry until it is translucent. Add the meat and cook until brown. Add in the seasoning and the tomato paste. Mix well and add the water in. Allow the sauce to come to a rolling boil, reduce the temperature and let it simmer for about 15 minutes or so, until the water has pretty much all cooked out. Take off the heat. Make the pasta sheets as follows: Set your oven at 300. Mix together the cream cheese, salt and eggs until it is completely smooth. Add the psyllium husks a small amount at a time until completely combined. Allow the mixture to rest for about five minutes. Grease a large baking tin and line with baking paper. Spread out the mixture nice and evenly. If necessary, roll out the batter so that it is thin enough and is 13 inches by 18 inches.

If you prefer to use a thinner pasta, divide it in two before rolling it out. Put in the oven and bake the pasta for around ten minutes or so. Set it aside to cool. Take it off the paper and then cut up into sheets. Set your oven at 400. Mix together the cheese, the cream and a large proportion of the Parmesan. Reserve a bit to sprinkle over the top of the lasagna. Season as you like and add the parsley. Grease an oven-proof dish Layer the sauce and pasta sheets into it. Top off with the cream mix and sprinkle with the leftover Parmesan. Bake for around half an hour or until it is completely warmed through and golden on top.

13. Your Keto BLT

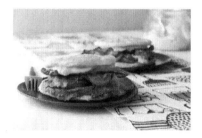

Serves 4

Ingredients

- 6 – 8 tablespoons mayo
- 8 pieces of bread (Recipe underneath)
- 4¾ ounces of bacon

- Freshly picked basil
- 1 tomato, sliced up nice and thin
- Lettuce

Ingredients for Bread

- 4 ¼ ounces of cream cheese
- 3 eggs
- Salt to taste
- ½ teaspoon baking powder
- ½ tablespoon powdered psyllium

Method

Bread: Separate the eggs. Whisk the whites with a little salt until they form stiff peaks. Mix the yolks with the cream cheese. Add the psyllium husks with the baking powder. Fold the yolks and whites together gently to retain the air. Grease a baking sheet and line with baking paper. Drop the batter onto the sheet to make eight different breads. Set your over at 300. Put in the center of your oven. Bake for around 20-25 minutes or until golden.

Building Sandwich: Set your stove to Med-High and fry your bacon until crispy. Put your bread out and top with about a tablespoon or two of mayo. Layer up the tomato and lettuce, with the chopped basil and the bacon. Close off the sandwich with another slice of bread.

14. Stuffed Mushrooms

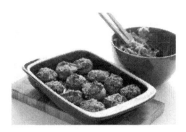

Serves 4

Ingredients

- 8 ounces of bacon
- 12 – 16 mushrooms
- 1 – 2 tablespoons farm butter
- 3 tablespoons fresh chives, chopped up nice and finely
- 7 ounces of cream cheese
- 1 teaspoon powdered paprika
- Seasoning to taste

Method

Set your oven at 400. Fry up the bacon until it is properly crisped. Set aside to cool and them crumble. Clean and chop the stems mushrooms up nice and finely, reserve the mushroom caps. Using the bacon fat, fry the mushrooms. If there is not enough grease, add the farm butter. Grease an oven-proof dish and put the mushrooms into it. Get a clean bowl and mix together all of the ingredients aside from the mushroom caps. Line up the mushroom caps in a single layer in the dish and divide the mixture evenly between all of them. Place in the oven uncovered and cook until the mushrooms start to get golden – around about 20 minutes.

15. Cheesy Meat Balls

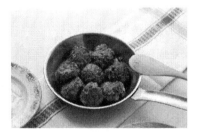

Serves 4

Ingredients

- 1 lot of pimiento cheese

- 1 ½ pounds beef, minced
- 2 tablespoons farm butter, to fry the food in
- Seasoning to taste

Method

Mix together the cheese and pimiento. Divide the meat into eight equal portions. Set the stove to Medium and then melt the farm butter in a heavy-based frying pan. Cook the meatballs in the butter and serve hot. Top with homemade mayo and serve with a leafy salad.

16. Zucchini Salad

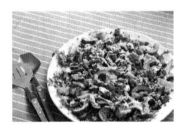

Serves 2

Ingredients

- 1 tablespoon olive oil
- 2 zucchinis
- Seasoning to taste
- ¾ cup chopped nuts of your choice
- 3 ½ ounces of arugula
- 1 head of romaine
- 5 1/3 tablespoons freshly picked chives

Ingredients for Dressing

- ¾ cup mayo
- ½ teaspoon table salt
- 2 tablespoons olive oil

- 1 garlic clove
- ¼ teaspoon chili powder

Method

Blend together all the ingredients for the dressing, which will give the flavor time to develop. Prepare the salad by splitting the zucchini length-wise, scoop out the seeds and slice crosswise. Trim and cut the salad. Place in a big bowl. Stir in the arugula lettuce and sprinkle the chives on top. Fry the zucchini quickly in olive oil until it has turned a nice color, it should stay firm. Seasoning to taste. Roast the nuts briefly in the same pan. Apply the zucchini and nuts on top of the green salad and pour dressing over it. Serve immediately as it is or with fried or grilled meat, chicken or fish.

17. Spicy Avocado Pie

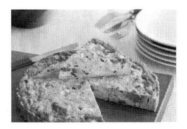

Serves 4-6

Ingredients for Pie crust

- 4 tablespoons Sesame seeds
- ¾ cup almond flour
- 4 tablespoons coconut flour
- 1 teaspoon baking powder
- 1 tablespoon powdered psyllium husks
- 1 pinch salt
- 4 tablespoons water
- 1 egg
- 3 tablespoons olive oil or coconut oil

Ingredients for Filling

- 1 cup mayo
- 2 ripe avocados
- 3 eggs
- 1 red chili pepper, chopped up nice and finely
- 2 tablespoons fresh cilantro, chopped up nice and finely
- 1¼ cups cheese, grated
- ½ teaspoon onion powder
- 8 tablespoons cream cheese
- ¼ teaspoon table salt

Method

Set your oven at 350. Put all the dough ingredients into your food processor or just combine with your hands – you want the dough to form up nice and firmly. Grease a 12-inch pie tin and cover the bottom with baking paper cut to size. Place the dough into the pie plate and then spread out so that it is evenly spaced across the bottom and the sides. Put the crust in the oven and bake for about 15 minutes. Peel the avocado and dice into small cubes. Mix these with the remaining ingredients and pour the new mixture into the pie crust. Put it in the oven for around 25 minutes or until it looks golden. Allow it to rest for a little before you serve. It can be served hot or cold.

18. Italian Style Pizza

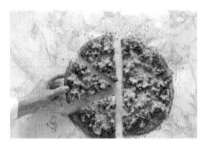

Serves 4

Ingredients for Dough

- ¾ cup almond flour
- 1½ cups grated mozzarella
- 2 tablespoons cream cheese
- 1 egg
- 1 teaspoon white wine vinegar
- olive oil to grease your hands
- ½ teaspoon table salt

Ingredients for Topping

- 1 tablespoon farm butter
- ½ pound Italian sausages
- ½ cup unsweetened tomato sauce
- 1½ cups grated mozzarella cheese
- ½ teaspoon dried oregano

Method

Set your oven at 400. Set your stove to Medium. Place the cream cheese and the mozzarella into a little, non-stick pot. Warm up and stir until they have melted together. Take off the heat and add in the remaining ingredients. Mix them well until you have a firm dough. Set the dough out on a silicon baking sheet or piece of baking paper. Flatten the dough until if forms a circle with an 8-inch diameter. You can use a rolling pin to flatten out the dough if you put a sheet of baking paper on top of it. Lay the crust out onto a greased baking tray. Prick the dough all over using a fork. Bake as is for around ten minutes or until it becomes golden.

In the meantime, set your stove to Medium and melt the farm butter in the pan. Add the sausage meat and stir well until done. Spread the top of the base with the tomato sauce. Put the remaining toppings on the pizza, ending with the cheese. Bake for about 10 minutes or until the cheese bubbles.

19. Chicken Curry

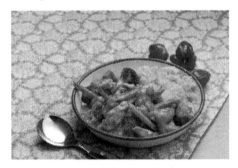

Serves 4

Ingredients

- ½ pound broccoli
- 1 pound chicken thighs, boneless
- 1 mild onion, chopped up nice and finely
- 3½ ounces of fresh green beans
- 2 cans coconut cream or coconut milk
- 3 tablespoons farm butter or coconut oil
- Seasoning to taste
- 1 tablespoon curry paste
- 1 tablespoon grated fresh ginger
- 1 red chili pepper, chopped up nice and finely or grated

Ingredients for Cauliflower Rice

- ½ teaspoon table salt
- 12/3 pounds cauliflower
- ½ teaspoon turmeric (optional)
- 3¼ ounces of farm butter or coconut oil

Method

Set your stove to Medium-High and put a pan on the plate. Add the coconut oil or butter and heat it up. Add the onion, chili and ginger and fry for a bit. Put the curry paste in and the fry up the chicken until lightly browned all over. If necessary, add more farm butter/ oil. Chop up the beans and broccoli and put them into your pan. Put in the coconut cream and season to taste. Reduce the heat to Low and allow the mixture to simmer until it is thick and creamy, stirring every once in a while.

Cauliflower Rice: Grate up the whole of the cauliflower. Set the stove at Medium and put the farm butter in a heavy-based skillet. Fry up the "rice" until it has softened up. Season to taste and the turmeric, if you are using it. Alternatively, you can do the "rice" in your microwave. Place it into a glass bowl and put plastic wrap over the top of it. Microwave it for about five minutes or until cooked through. Mix together with the farm butter and serve.

20. Fish Pie for Adults

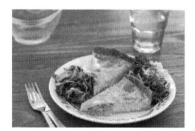

Serves 4-6

Ingredients for Pie Crust

- 4 tablespoons Sesame seeds
- ¾ cup almond flour
- 4 tablespoons coconut flour
- 1 teaspoon baking powder
- 1 tablespoon powdered psyllium husks
- 1 pinch salt
- 4 tablespoons water
- 1 egg
- 3 tablespoons olive oil or coconut oil

Ingredients for Filling

- 1 cup mayo
- ½ pound smoked salmon
- 3 eggs
- ½ teaspoon onion powder
- 2 tablespoons fresh dill, chopped up nice and finely
- ¼ teaspoon powdered black pepper
- 1¼ cups cheese, grated
- 4¼ ounces of cream cheese

Method

Set your oven at 350. Mix up the crust ingredients so that they form a firm dough. Grease a 10-inch pie tin and line it with baking paper. Spread out the dough on top so that it covers the base of the pie tin and the sides. Make sure that it's evenly spread out. Put the crust in the oven and bake for 15 minutes. In the meanwhile, mix together all the ingredients for the topping, barring the salmon. Add to the pie crust and top off with the salmon. Put in the oven for about half an hour or until your pie looks nice and golden. Allow it to cool a little before serving.

21. Low-Carb Frittata with Fresh Spinach

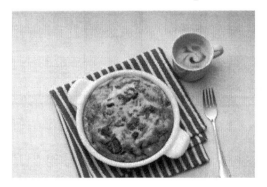

Serves 4

Ingredients

- 1 cup double cream
- 8 eggs
- ½ pound fresh spinach
- 1/3 pound cheese, grated
- Seasoning to taste
- 1/3 pound diced bacon or chorizo
- 2 tablespoons farm butter, for frying

Method

Set your oven at 350. Set your stove to Med-High and melt the farm butter. Add in the bacon and cook till nice and crisp. Stir in the spinach and let it wilt. Set aside. Grease an oven-proof dish. Whisk together the cream and eggs and pour into the dish. Put the spinach and bacon mixture and top off with the cheese. Put onto the middle rack in your oven and bake for around a half an hour or so.

22. Mushroom and Bacon Pierogis

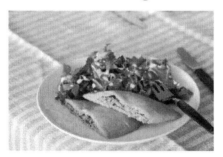

Serves 4

Ingredients for Filling

- 2 garlic cloves, chopped up nice and finely
- 2 tablespoons farm butter
- 1 shallot, chopped up nice and finely
- 2 ounces of bacon

- 3¼ ounces of mushrooms
- 2 ounces of fresh spinach
- 1/3 pound cream cheese
- ¼ teaspoon pepper
- 2 ounces of Parmesan, grated
- ½ teaspoon table salt

Ingredients for the Dough

- 2 2/3 ounces of farm butter
- 4 tablespoons coconut flour
- 8 tablespoons almond flour
- ½ teaspoon table salt
- 1½ cups cheese, grated
- 1 teaspoon baking powder
- 1 beaten egg, for brushing the top
- 1 egg

Method

Make the filling first. Set the stove to Med-High and heat the farm butter in a heavy-based frying pan. Add the garlic, shallots, mushrooms, spinach and bacon and cook through. Season to taste. Set the heat to Med-Low and mix in the cheeses. Mix well and allow the mixture to simmer for a minute or so. Put to one side so that it can cool off. Set your oven at 350. Now you can make the dough. Put all the dry ingredients into a large bowl and mix it up. Set your stove to Low and let the butter melt in a heavy-based frying pan. Add the cheese, stirring continuously, so that you have a nice lump-free batter. Take off the stove. Add an egg to the mixture while still stirring. Stir in the dry mixture until you have made a firm dough. The dough should then be divided into four equally-sized balls. Flatten them out so that they are around 1/5th inch thick and circular in shape. Divide the filling up between the rolled-out dough. Take care to cover only half of the dough. You can then fold up the other side so that you can seal the pierogis. Beat an egg and brush the top of the dough with it. Place the pierogis onto a greased baking tray and serve warm.

23. Salad in A Jar

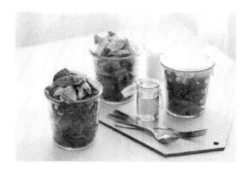

Serves 1

Ingredients

- 1 ounce of leafy greens
- 4 ounces of cooked meat of your choice – this is a great way to use up leftovers
- 1 ounce of cherry tomatoes
- 1 ounce of cucumber
- 4 tablespoons mayo or olive oil
- 1 ounce of red bell peppers
- 1 ounce of carrots, grated
- ½ scallion

Method

Chop up all the veggies that you are using until they are in bite-sized pieces. Get a clean mason jar and put a layer of the leafy greens in first. You can also, if you prefer, make this a layer of finely chopped cauliflower or broccoli. Layer the other ingredients = the onions, carrot, bell peppers and the cherry tomatoes. Finish it off with the meat of your choice. Alternatively, you can switch this out for other protein such as tuna, hard-boiled eggs, nuts, cheese, etc. Keep the mayo or dressing into a different container and serve the salad with that.

24. Quesadillas

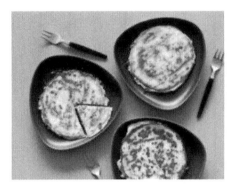

Serves 3

Ingredients

- 1 teaspoon olive oil for frying
- 1/3 pound cheese, grated
- 6 low-carb tortillas
- 1 ounces of leafy greens

Ingredients for Low-Carb Tortillas

- ½ teaspoon table salt
- 2 egg whites
- 2 eggs
- 6 ounces of cream cheese
- 1 tablespoon coconut flour
- 1 – 2 teaspoons powdered psyllium husks

Method

Tortillas: Set your oven at 400. Whisk up the egg whites and the eggs until they start to froth up. Whisk in the cream cheese as well so that everything is combined well. In a different bowl, mix together the psyllium, salt and coconut flour until completely combine. Add the dry mix a little at a time to the cream cheese mix. You want the batter to be smooth and thick. Grease two baking tins and line them with baking paper. Pour the batter out onto the sheets, creating six different rounds for the tortillas. Spread the batter out so that it is no more than a quarter inch thick. Put on the uppermost rack in the oven and bake for four or five minutes. The tortillas are done when they start to turn brown.

Quesadillas: Set out half the tortillas onto a big cutting board. Divide half of the cheese up between the tortillas. Layer on the greens, put the rest of the cheese over the top. Finish them off with the remaining tortillas. Set your stove to Med-High. Heat some farm butter up in a heavy-bottomed frying pan and add the quesadillas. Cook for around about a minute and flip. Cook for another minute. You want the cheese to melt here.

25. Mushroom and Cheese omelet

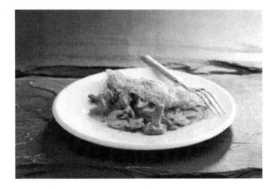

Serves 1

Ingredients

- 7/8 ounces of farm butter, for frying
- 3 eggs
- 7/8 ounces of cheese, grated
- 2 – 3 mushrooms, chopped up nice and finely
- 1/4 mild onion, chopped up nice and finely
- Seasoning to taste

Method

Beat the eggs well and season to taste. Add the spices you are using. Set your stove to Medium and melt the farm butter in a heavy-based frying pan. Add the eggs and let them cook until nearly done. Add the onion, mushrooms and cheese on top. Take your spatula and use to fold the omelet. Serve it straight away.

26. Spicy Indian Chicken

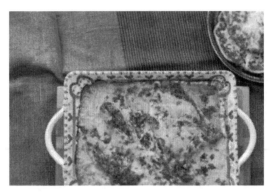

Serves 6-8

Ingredients

- 3 tablespoons farm butter
- 23 ounces of chicken breasts
- salt
- 1 tablespoon freshly picked parsley, chopped up nice and finely
- 1¼ cups sour cream or double cream
- 1 red bell pepper, finely diced

Ingredients for Garam Masala

- 1 – 2 teaspoons coriander seeds, ground
- 1 teaspoon powdered cumin
- 1 teaspoon ground cardamom

- 1 teaspoon ground ginger
- 1 teaspoon turmeric, ground
- 1 teaspoon paprika powder
- 1 pinch ground nutmeg
- ½ – 1 teaspoon chili powder

Method

Set your oven at 400. Slice up the chicken into evenly sized strips and fry in some oil until the meat starts to brown. Divide the garam masala into two even portions and add one to the chicken. Season to taste. Grease an oven-proof dish and put the chicken into it. Pour the pan juices over the top. Mix together the cream, the pepper and the leftover portion of the garam masala. Pour over the top of the chicken. Put in the oven for around 20-25 minutes until all done.

27. Sausage and Broccoli Bake

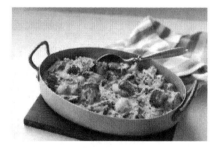

Serves 4-6

Ingredients

- 1 leek
- 1 pound sausages, cooked ahead of time
- 1 mild onion
- ½ pound cauliflower, cut up into florets
- 1 pound broccoli, cut up into florets
- 1 cup sour cream
- 2 tablespoons Dijon mustard

- 1¾ ounces of farm butter, for frying
- Seasoning to taste
- 4¼ ounces of cheese, grated
- 4 tablespoons fresh thyme

Method

Set your oven at 450. Chop up the onion and leek into coarse pieces. Do the same with the cauliflower and the broccoli. Cut up the sausages as well. Try and keep the pieces all about the same size. Set your stove to Medium and melt the farm butter. Put in the onions and fry until translucent. Add the rest of the vegetables and fry until they just start to soften a little. Grease an oven-proof dish and put the vegetables into it in one layer. Mix the cream and the mustard and pour the over the top of the veggies. Put the sausage on top, season with finely chopped thyme and top off with the cheese. Put on one of the upper racks of the oven for about 15 minutes or so. The cheese should be bubbly and the whole thing heated through.

28. Broccoli and Fish Oven Bake

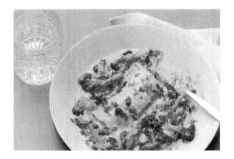

Serves 4

Ingredients

- 1 pound broccoli
- 2 tablespoons olive oil
- 6 scallions
- 1 ounce of farm butter, to grease the dish

- 2 tablespoons small capers
- 1½ pounds white fish, in bite-sized pieces
- 1 tablespoon Dijon mustard
- 1¼ cups double cream
- 3¼ ounces of farm butter
- 1 teaspoon table salt
- 1 tablespoon dried parsley
- ¼ teaspoon powdered black pepper

For serving

- 1/3 pound leafy greens

Method

Set your oven at 400. Cut the broccoli up into small pieces. Use the stem as well. Set the stove to Med-High and heat some oil in a heavy-based frying pan. Add the broccoli and fry until it softens up nicely. Season to taste. Chop up the scallions and capers finely. Add them to the pan and fry for around a minute or two. Grease an oven-proof dish, layer the veggies and fish in the dish. Mix together the cream, mustard and parsley and pour on top. Put in your oven and cook through until the fish is done. It will take around 20 minutes. This dish works well with a leafy green salad.

29. Beef Tortillas

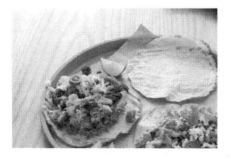

Serves 6

Ingredients

- 1½ pounds beef, minced
- 8 – 12 low-carb tortillas
- 2 tablespoons olive oil
- 1 teaspoon table salt
- 1 cup of plain
- grated leafy greens
- 1 – 1 2/3 cups cheese, grated

Ingredients for Salsa

- 1 – 2 tomatoes, chopped into small cubes
- 2 avocados, chopped into small cubes
- Seasoning to taste
- 8 tablespoons fresh cilantro, chopped
- 1 lime, the juice
- 1 tablespoon olive oil

Ingredients for Tex-Mex Seasoning

- 2 teaspoons paprika powder
- 2 teaspoons chili powder
- 1 teaspoon powdered cumin
- 1 pinch cayenne pepper
- 1 – 2 teaspoons mild onions or garlic powder
- Seasoning to taste

Method

Set the stove to Med-High. Warm up the oil in a heavy-based saucepan and fry up the mince until it is nicely browned. Season to taste and add the taco seasoning along with the water. Bring it to the boil. Reduce the heat to Low and cook, stirring every once in a while, until the liquid has cooked out. Now you can make the salsa. Mix together all the ingredients for the salsa. Season as you like. Put some lettuce into the tortillas, spoon some of the mince in as well and top with the cheese. Serve the salsa on the side.

30. Shepherd's Pie Rebooted

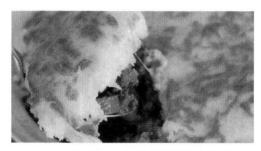

Serves 8

Ingredients for the Filling

- 1 mild onion diced
- 3 carrots finely grated
- Extra virgin olive oil
- 1 pound of mince
- 13 ounces of canned tomatoes, chopped up
- 2 cloves garlic crushed
- 1/4 cup beef stock

Ingredients for the Topping

- 50g / 1/2 stick butter
- A cauliflower that is on the small side, grated coarsely
- 2tbsp heavy cream
- ½ cup grated Cheddar
- Seasoning to taste

Method

Set your oven to 350. Start by making the filling. Set your stove to Med-High and warm up the oil in a heavy=based saucepan. Put the garlic and the onion into the saucepan and cook until it is just starting to soften. Put your mince into the saucepan and cook until it is browned and cooked throughout. Add the tomatoes, the carrots and the stock. Stir well and bring to the boil. Reduce the heat to Low and let the mixture simmer while you prepare the topping. It should cook for about 10 minutes or so, until all the liquid cooks out, without the lid on. You should stir once in a while.

The Topping: Boil up the cauliflower until it is done. It will be about ten minutes. Drain well and ensure that there is no steam left in the pot. Mix together the cream, seasoning and the butter. Puree the mixture until it resembles mashed potatoes. Grease an oven-proof dish and layer the mince into an even layer in the dish. Put the mash on top and finish with a layer of cheese. Put the dish into the oven and bake for about half an hour.

31. Pizza with A Twist

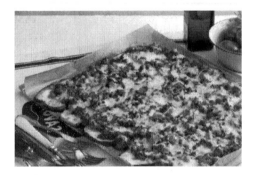

Serves 4

Ingredients

- 1/3 olive oil to brush on or to fry
- 2 eggplants
- 2 garlic cloves
- ¾ pound beef, minced
- 1 mild onion
- 7 ounces of tomato sauce

- ¼ cup chopped fresh oregano
- ½ teaspoon pepper
- 1 teaspoon table salt
- 2/3 pound cheese, grated
- ½ teaspoon powdered cinnamon, powdered (optional)

Method

Set your oven at 400. Cut the eggplants into rings about a half inch thick. Brush on some olive oil and put in an oven-proof dish in the oven. Cook for about 15-20 minutes or until they start to go golden. Chop the garlic up nice and finely, and do the same with the onion. Set your stove to Medium and put some oil in a pan. Fry the onion and garlic until they start to turn translucent. Put your meat into the pan and cook until lightly brown. Season to taste and then add in the tomato, oregano and cinnamon. Reduce the heat to Low and let it simmer for about 10 or 15 minutes. Layer the meat mixture on top of the eggplant, and make a mini-pizza from each slice. Add a sprinkling of oregano and cheese. Bake for another 10 minutes or till the cheese is bubbling.

32. Cauliflower and Artichoke Pizza

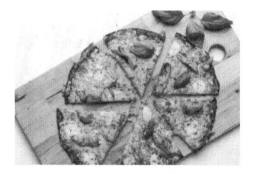

Serves 2-3

Ingredients

- 4¾ ounces cauliflower, grated coarsely
- ½ teaspoon table salt

- 3½ ounces of cheese, grated
- 2 eggs

Ingredients for Toppings

- 1¾ ounces of cheese, grated
- 1 garlic clove, sliced up nice and finely
- 4 tablespoons tomato sauce
- 1 tablespoon dried oregano
- 1 – 2 canned artichokes, cut into wedges
- 2 ounces of Mozzarella

Method

Set your oven at 350. Put the cauliflower into a large bowl and mix in the eggs and cheese. Grease a baking sheet and line it with baking paper. Spread it out in a thin layer in an 11-inch circle. Put in the oven and let it cook for around 15-20 minutes or so. Take out of the oven and let it cool down a little. Spread out the tomato sauce in an even layer. Put on the artichokes on top and also add the garlic if you like. Add the oregano and sprinkle with the cheese. Set your oven at 420 and put it back in the oven. Cook it until the cheese starts to bubble.

33. Pizza Made from Tortillas

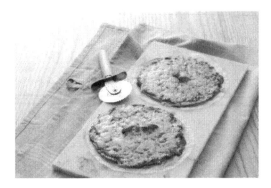

Serves 4

Ingredients

- 4 – 6 low-carb tortillas

Ingredients for Topping

- 2 cups cheese, grated
- 8 tablespoons tomato sauce
- Seasoning to taste
- 1 – 2 teaspoons dried oregano

Method

Set your oven at 450. Put about a tablespoon or two of the tomato paste onto each of the tortillas and spread it out evenly. Season to taste and top off with cheese. Cook until the cheese bubbles.

34. Peperoni Pizza

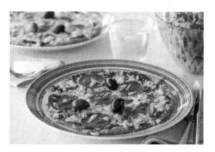

Serves 4

Ingredients for the Crust

- 6¼ ounces of Mozzarella, grated
- 4 eggs

Ingredients for the Topping

- 1 teaspoon dried oregano
- 4 tablespoons tomato paste

- 4¼ ounces of Cheddar, grated
- Olives to taste
- 1¾ ounces of pepperoni

For serving

- Table salt
- Olive oil
- 1/3 pound leafy greens

Method

Set your oven at 400. To make the crust, beat together the egg and Mozzarella. Grease a baking tray and line with baking paper. Create two pizza bases out of the batter and spread them out thinly on the paper. Put in the oven and cook until it starts to become a little golden. It will be 10-15 minutes. Take out and set aside so that it can cool off a bit. Set your oven to 450. Divide the tomato paste evenly between the bases and put some oregano on it. Slice up the olives and sprinkle over the pizza and then top with pepperoni and the Cheddar. Put in the oven and cook until the cheese starts bubbling.

35. Pizza Entrees

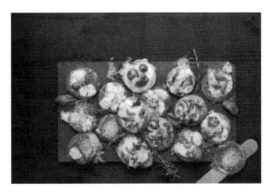

Serves 4

Ingredients for the Crust

- 5 1/3 tablespoons mayo
- 3 eggs
- 3 tablespoons coconut flour
- ½ teaspoon table salt
- 1 tablespoon olive oil
- 1 teaspoon baking powder
- ½ teaspoon onion powder

Ingredients for the Toppings

- 1 teaspoon table salt
- 8 tablespoons tomato paste
- Toppings of your choice – olives, tomatoes, shrimps, sausage
- ¼ teaspoon powdered black pepper
- 2 ounces of fresh Parmesan, grated
- ½ pound Mozzarella, grated
- 1 tablespoon olive oil

Method

Whisk up the eggs and add the mayo until incorporated. In a separate bowl, mix all the dry ingredients together. Fold the egg mix in carefully until there are no lumps. Set the stove to Med-High and heat up enough oil to cover the bottom of a heavy-bottomed frying pan. Spoon the mixture into the frying pan, making 3-inch circles. Cook until golden on either side. Line a baking sheet with baking paper and place the bases onto it. Set your oven at 400. Spoon some of the tomato base onto each pizza in an even layer and top with whatever toppings you like. Add some oregano and seasoning as required. Finish off with a layer of cheese. Place in the oven and cook until the cheese is bubbling.

36. Tuna Melt

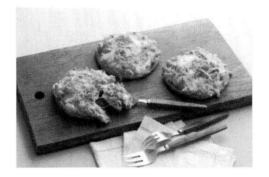

Serves 3

Ingredients for the Salad

- 4 celery stalks
- 1 cup mayo or sour cream
- ½ cup pickles, chopped
- 1 teaspoon lemon juice
- 2 cans tuna packed in olive oil
- Seasoning to taste
- 1 garlic clove, minced

Ingredients for the Toppings

- ¼ teaspoon cayenne
- 2/3 pound cheese, grated

For Serving

- olive oil
- 1/3 pound leafy greens

Bread for The Sandwiches (makes 8)

- 4¼ ounces of cream cheese
- 3 eggs

- 1 pinch salt
- ½ teaspoon baking powder
- ½ tablespoon powdered psyllium husks

Method

Set your oven at 300. Mix together the ingredients for the salad.

Make the bread next: Separate the egg whites and yolks and place them in different bowls. Whip up the whites with the salt until they become stiff peaks. Beat up the yolks and the cream cheese. Add in the psyllium seed husks, along with the baking powder and mix until completely incorporated. Fold the two egg mixes together, being gentle so as not to lose the air in the whites. Grease a baking tin and line it with baking paper. Divide the bread mix into 8 equal portions and put onto the baking tray. Put in the oven on the center rack. Cook for around 25 minutes or until they brown nicely. Remove the bread and replace the baking paper. Lay out the breads on the sheet again and spoon on the salad mix. Season to taste and add the Cayenne. Add cheese. Bake until the cheese is bubbling hot. Serve with a green salad.

37. Chili Salmon with Leafy Greens

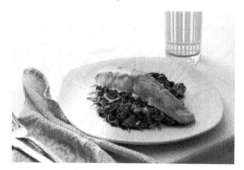

Serves 4

Ingredients

- 1 tablespoon chili paste
- 1½ pounds salmon, in pieces

- 1¾ ounces of farm butter or olive oil
- 1 cup mayo or sour cream
- 1 pound fresh spinach
- 4 tablespoons grated Parmesan

Method

Set your oven at 400. Start by seasoning the salmon as you want. Grease an oven-proof dish, with the skin side facing down. Mix together the chili paste, the mayo, and the cheese until properly combined and spread all over the salmon. Put in the oven for around 15 minutes or so until the fish is cooked. About 5 minutes before the fish is ready, set your stove to Med-High and melt the farm butter in a large frying pan or wok. Add the spinach, making sure it is evenly coated. Cook for a few minutes until the spinach wilts. Plate the spinach and serve the salmon on top of it.

Chapter 3: Dinner

1. Turkey Soup with An Asian Twist

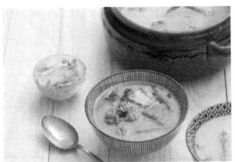

Serves 4

Ingredients for Turkey Soup

- 1 mild onion
- 3 tablespoons coconut oil
- 1 ounces of fresh ginger, peeled and grated

- 1 tablespoon green curry paste
- 27 ounces of coconut milk
- 1 pound ground turkey
- 2 cups water
- 1 bell pepper of your choice
- 2 teaspoons salt
- 4 ounces of fresh green beans
- ½ teaspoon pepper

Farm Butter

- ⅓ cup chopped fresh cilantro
- 2 tablespoons olive oil
- 4 ounces of farm butter
- ½ teaspoon crushed coriander seeds
- 1 pinch pepper
- 1 teaspoon table salt
- 1 tablespoon lime juice

Method

Chop up the ginger and the onion. Set your stove to Med-High and heat up the oil in a heavy-based frying pan. When hot, stir in the onion and cook until they start to turn translucent. Stir in the turkey and fry, stirring regularly, until the turkey is done. Mix in the pepper and the curry paste. Put everything else that is left, aside from the beans, into the beans. Allow the mixture to come to a boil. Reduce the heat to Low and allow the mixture to cook for around 20 minutes. Clean the beans and chop up roughly. When the soup has been on for around 10 minutes, put the beans in the soup. Serve with the butter.

For the Butter: Mix together the cilantro and the oil. Blend with the butter until the butter becomes creamy.

2. Tangy Ham with Fruit

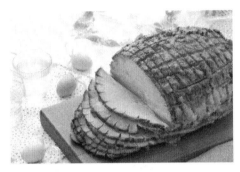

Serves 12

Ingredients

- Water
- 5 pounds whole ham, pre-cooked and properly cured

Glaze

- 3 tablespoons Dijon mustard
- 3 ounces of apricots, dried
- 1 teaspoon table salt
- 1 teaspoon ground allspice (if you like)
- 2 tablespoons olive oil
- 1 teaspoon tabasco

Method

The night before you are going to prepare this meal, cover the apricots in enough water to completely submerge them and set aside. The next morning, drain off any remaining water and chop the apricots nice and finely. Puree the apricots and the remaining ingredients for the glaze. Set your oven at 350. Cut the top of the ham so that you have a grid of squares. Grease a roasting tin and fill it about half way so that there is plenty of water to keep the ham moist during cooking. Brush the ham with the glaze and put it into the oven. Cook for around 1.5 – 2 hours. The cooking time depends on the size of the ham. The idea here is not to recook the meat but to get the glaze to caramelize. Check that the ham is completely heated by measuring the temperature at the thickest portion of your ham. The thermometer should read 120. If you feel that the ham is begging too dry, you can place some foil over the top. Serve hot or cold, in nice thin slices.

3. Buttery Broccoli

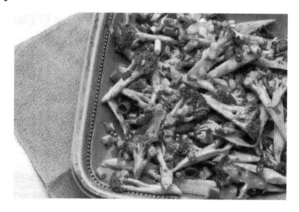

Serves 4

Ingredients

- 1 pound broccoli
- 3¼ ounces of farm butter
- 5 scallions
- Seasoning to taste
- 2 tablespoons small capers (optional)

Method

Chop up the broccoli into small pieces. Cut up the stem in the same way. Set your stove to Med-High and melt the farm butter. Add the broccoli and stir to coat with the butter. Cook for around 5-10 minutes or until the broccoli is just done. Season as required. Chop up the scallions and the capers. Stir in the capers and scallions. Fry for a couple more minutes.

4. Tenderloin and Mash

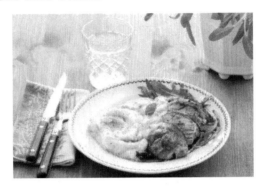

Serves 4

Ingredients for the Tenderloin

- 7 ounces of bacon
- 1 1/3 pounds pork tenderloin
- ½ teaspoon pepper
- 1 tablespoon olive oil
- 1 tablespoon farm butter
- 1/3 pound cream cheese
- 1 ounce of sun-dried tomatoes, chopped
- 1 garlic clove, minced
- 2 tablespoons fresh sage, chopped up nice and finely
- ¾ cup double cream
- Seasoning to taste

Ingredients for the Mash

- 1 whole garlic bulb
- 1 tablespoon olive oil
- Seasoning to taste
- ½ teaspoon table salt
- 4 ounces of farm butter
- 1 pound cauliflower

Method

Start by preparing the mash. Once it is done, place into a warmer drawer while preparing the rest of the food. Set the oven at 350. Mix together the tomatoes, cream cheese, sage and garlic. Season the tenderloin and cut a pocket running through it lengthwise. Spoon in around about half the filling and then close it as best you can. Wrap in the bacon. Set your stove to Med-High. Place the olive oil and butter into a heavy-based frying pan. Brown the tenderloin/ bacon. Grease an oven-proof dish and place the tenderloin in it. Place the tenderloin into the oven. The pork is cooked when your meat thermometer reads 150. It is best to use the meat thermometer so that you know when the meat is done. Wrap the tenderloin in a foil tent and put aside to rest. Set your stove to Medium and put the pan juices into the frying pan that you browned the meat in. Stir in the remaining filling ingredients and allow to come to a gentle boil. Reduce the temperature to Low and allow it to simmer for about five minutes. Season as required.

Make the Mash: Set your oven at 425. Break up the cloves but do not peel them. Put it into an oven-safe dish and drizzle the olive oil over it. Season as required. Cook for about 20-30 minutes or until the garlic softens. In the meantime, clean the cauliflower and chop it up finely. Set your stove to Med-High. Place the cauliflower in a pot and cover with water. Salt the water as required and cook until it soft. Drain the cauliflower well, get as much of the water out as you can. Remove the garlic peel and blend it with the cauliflower and the farm butter. Adjust the seasoning as required.

5. Chicken with Tomato-Flavored Farm butter

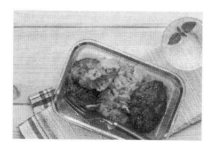

Serves 4

Ingredients for the Chicken

- 1 egg
- 1⅓ pounds ground chicken
- ½ mild onion, chopped up nice and finely
- ½ teaspoon powdered black pepper
- 1 teaspoon table salt
- 2 ounces of farm butter, to use for frying
- 1 teaspoon dried thyme

Ingredients for the Cabbage

- ½ teaspoon powdered black pepper
- 3 ounces of farm butter
- 1½ pounds cabbage
- 1 teaspoon table salt

Ingredients for the Tomato-Flavored Butter

- 1 tablespoon tomato paste
- Seasoning to taste
- 4 ounces of farm butter
- 1 teaspoon red wine vinegar

Method

Set your oven at 220°F. Blend together each of the ingredients for the chicken and divide into 8 evenly-sized patties. Set your stove to Med-High and melt the farm butter in a heavy-based frying pan. Put the patties in and fry for few minutes on each side until done. Remove and put in a warmer drawer. Coarsely grate the cabbage and put into the frying pan that you cooked the patties in. Set your stove to Med-High and fry the cabbage until it is brown and caramelized. Season as required. Put the ingredients for the butter and beat it until everything is combined. Plate the cabbage and serve the chicken with a pat of the butter.

6. Pastrami Salad

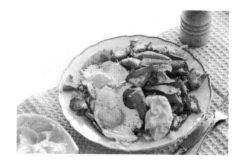

Serves 2

Ingredients

- 2 tablespoons Dijon mustard
- 8 tablespoons mayo
- 1 shallot
- 4 ounces of lettuce
- 1 dill pickle
- ½ pound pastrami
- 4 low-carb croutons with Parmesan
- 4 eggs

Method

Mix the mustard and the mayo together and put to one side. Plate the lettuce. Chop your onion up nice and finely and add to the lettuce. Do the same with the cucumber. Top with your pastrami and the mustard mayo to taste. Cook the eggs to your liking, right before you are ready to serve. Place the eggs on the salad and sprinkle the croutons on top.

7. Avocado and Egg Cabbage Salad

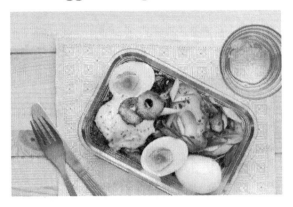

Serves 2

Ingredients

- 1 tablespoon Dijon mustard
- ½ cup mayo
- 4 eggs
- 3 ounces of kale
- ½ pound broccoli
- Seasoning to taste
- 1 ounce of scallions
- 2 garlic cloves
- 2 tablespoons olive oil
- 2 avocados
- 1 pinch chili flakes

Method

Stir the mustard and the mayo together and put to one side. Cook the eggs to your likely and peel them. Halve eggs and set aside. Peel the avocado and remove the pit. Chop into thin slices. Set your stove to Medium and warm the oil in a heavy-based frying pan. Crush the garlic and fry it for about a minute. Remove it from the frying pan. Chop the kale and broccoli up nice and finely. Place into the frying pan that you cooked the garlic in. Stir well to coat with the oil and fry until just done. Season to taste. Plate all the food.

8. Pork Skewers and Mash

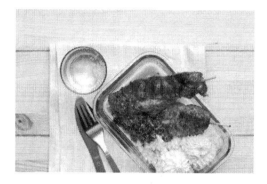

Serves 4

Ingredients for Pork Skewers

- 1 tablespoon farm butter
- ½ tablespoon Ranch seasoning
- 1 pound pork shoulders, cut into bite-sized pieces
- 1 teaspoon table salt

Ingredients for the Mash

- Seasoning as required
- ⅓ pound farm butter
- 23 ounces of cauliflower
- 2 ounces of grated Parmesan

Ingredients for Salsa Verde

- 3⅓ tablespoons freshly picked cilantro, chopped up nice and finely
- 6¾ tablespoons freshly picked parsley, chopped up nice and finely
- 2 garlic cloves, crushed

- 3 1/3 tablespoons small capers
- The juice of ½ lemon
- 2/3 cup olive oil
- ½ teaspoon powdered black pepper
- 1 teaspoon table salt

Method

Start by making the sauce. Take all the sauce ingredients and blend until smooth. Coat the meat with the Ranch seasoning and then thread it onto the skewers. Set your stove to Medium and melt the farm butter in a heavy-based frying pan that is big enough to fit the skewers in. Cook for a few minutes on each side until the chicken is done throughout. Set aside in the warmer drawer and move on to making the mash. Chop the cauliflower up nice and finely. Put the cauliflower in a pot with enough water to completely submerge it and season to taste. Set your stove to High and cook the cauliflower until it is tender. Drain off as much of the water as you can and blend the cauliflower into a puree, along with the farm butter and the cheese. Adjust the seasoning if you need to and serve.

9. Pork Chops

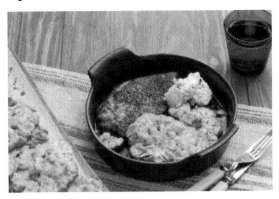

Serves 4

Ingredients for Herbed Farm butter

- 1 garlic clove
- 4 ounces of farm butter, softened
- 1 teaspoon lemon juice
- Seasoning to taste
- 1/3 cup freshly picked parsley, chopped up nice and finely

Pork Chops

- 2 ounces of farm butter, to fry the chops in
- 1 tablespoon Ranch seasoning
- 4 pork shoulder chops

Cauliflower

- 3 ounces of fresh Parmesan, grated
- 2 tablespoons olive oil
- 1½ pounds cauliflower

Method

Set your oven at 400. Get started with the herbed farm butter. Cream the butter and mix with the other ingredients until combined. Put to one side. Cook the cauliflower next. Break it up a bit, cutting in halves or quarters if necessary. Grease a baking tin and line it with baking paper. Lay the cauliflower on the tin in one layer. Brush the olive oil onto each surface of the cauliflower and season as you like. Sprinkle the Parmesan over the top and place in the oven for about 25 minutes or until cooked through and nicely brown outside. While the cauliflower is roasting, set your stove to Med-High and prepare the chops. Melt the butter in a heavy-based frying pan, season the chops to taste and cook or around 5 minutes per side or until cooked throughout. Set aside to rest for a little before serving.

10. Nasi Goreng

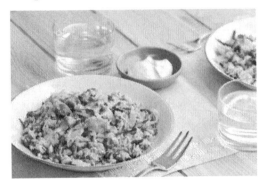

Serves 2

Ingredients for Lime Dressing

- The juice and zest of ½ lime
- ½ cup mayo

Ingredients for Nasi Goreng

- ½ mild onion
- 1 pound cauliflower
- 2 ounces of scallions
- 1 chili pepper
- ½ bell pepper of your choice
- 4 ounces of farm butter
- 1 ounces of fresh ginger, peeled and grated
- 2 garlic cloves, crushed
- 1 tablespoon Sesame oil
- Seasoning to taste
- 4 eggs

Method

Start with the dressing. Mix together the ingredients and put to one side. Grate up the cauliflower coarsely. Chop the onion, pepper and chili until nice and fine. Set your stove to Med-High and heat up the butter in a heavy-based frying pan. Stir in the veggies. Cook until almost done, adding the ginger and the garlic when the other veggies are almost done. Season as you like. Crack each of the eggs into the pan and heat until just set. Stir in and cook until the eggs are done to your liking. Serve with the dressing on top.

11. Meatballs with Basil Sauce

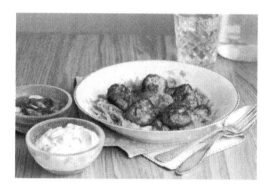

Serves 4

Ingredients

- ½ mild onion, chopped up nice and finely
- 1 1/3 pounds ground pork
- 1 tablespoon fresh ginger, peeled and grated
- 1 teaspoon powdered black pepper
- 1 tablespoon fish sauce
- 2 tablespoons coconut oil
- 2 ounces of farm butter or coconut oil
- 1 1/3 pounds cabbage

Ingredients for the Onion Salad

- 1 red chili pepper
- 1 tablespoon rice vinegar
- 1 ounce of scallions
- ½ teaspoon table salt

- 2 tablespoons water

Basil Sauce

- Seasoning to taste
- ¾ cup mayo
- 2 ounces of radishes
- ½ tablespoon freshly picked basil, chopped up nice and finely

Method

Start with the onion salad. Chop the scallions and pepper up nice and finely. Add in the vinegar, the salt and the water. Mix in with the scallions and chili and put aside to allow the flavors to develop. Move on to the Basil sauce. Chop up the radishes nice and finely and blend with the mayo and the basil. Season as you like and put to one side.

Make the meatballs now. Divide the meat into about 20 balls. Set your stove to Medium and warm the oil in a heavy-based frying pan. Add the meatballs and cook until done. Set aside and keep it warm. Coarsely grate the cabbage. Place in the same frying pan that you used to cook the meatballs, adding more butter if necessary. Set the stove to Med-High and stir-fry the cabbage until done. Serve straightaway.

12. Asian Cabbage Stir-Fry

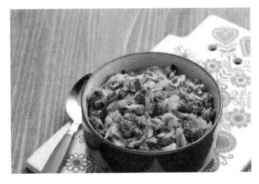

Serves 4

Ingredients

- 1/3 pound farm butter
- 1 2/3 pounds cabbage
- 1 1/3 pounds beef, minced
- 1 teaspoon onion powder
- 1 teaspoon table salt
- ¼ teaspoon powdered black pepper
- 2 garlic cloves
- 1 tablespoon white wine vinegar
- 1 tablespoon sesame oil
- 3 scallions, in slices
- 1 tablespoon fresh ginger, chopped up nice and finely or grated
- 1 teaspoon chili flakes

Wasabi mayo

- ½ – 1 tablespoon wasabi paste
- 1 cup mayo

Method

Coarsely grate the cabbage. Set stove to Med-High and melt the farm butter in a heavy-based frying pan. Stir in the cabbage and cook until just done. Mix together the vinegar and spices. Add it to the frying pan and fry for a little longer and set the cabbage to one side. Put some more farm butter into your pan. Fry the chili, ginger and garlic for a couple of minutes. Stir in the meat and cook until completely cooked, browned and there are no pan juices left. Reduce the heat. Mix together the cabbage and the scallions and heat until it warmed through. Drizzle the Sesame oil over the top just before you serve. Make the Wasabi mayo by adding small amounts of Wasabi to the mayo until you get the taste as you like.

13. Stir-Fried Cabbage

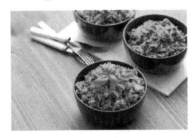

Serves 4

Ingredients

- 1/3 pound farm butter
- 1 2/3 pounds green cabbage
- 1 1/3 pounds beef, minced
- 1 teaspoon onion powder
- 1 teaspoon table salt
- ¼ teaspoon pepper
- 1 tablespoon tomato paste
- 1 cup sour cream
- 1 tablespoon white wine vinegar
- 3¼ ounces of leeks, chopped up nice and finely
- 2 garlic cloves, chopped up nice and finely
- 3 tablespoons fresh basil

Method

Coarsely grate the cabbage. Set your stove to Medium and melt the farm butter in a heavy-based frying pan. Stir in the cabbage and cook until softened. Put the vinegar and spices and stir in. Fry for a couple of minutes and then set aside. Using the same pan, heat up some more farm butter and stir in the leeks and garlic. Cook for a minute or so. Stir in the meat and fry until cooked completely and the pan juices have mostly cooked out. Mix in the tomato paste and reduce the heat. Stir in the cabbage and the basil. Heat until heated through. Season as you like and serve with sour cream.

14. Cheesy Stir-Fried Cabbage

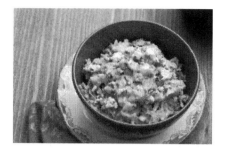

Serves 4

Ingredients

- ⅓ pound farm butter
- 1⅔ pounds green cabbage
- 1⅓ pounds beef, minced
- 1 teaspoon onion powder
- 1 teaspoon table salt
- ¼ teaspoon powdered black pepper
- 1 tablespoon white wine vinegar
- 2 teaspoons dried thyme
- 1 cup double cream
- 8 tablespoons freshly picked parsley, chopped up nice and finely
- ⅓ pound blue cheese

Method

Grate the cabbage as finely as possible. Set the stove to Med-High. Add about 2 ounces of the farm butter to a wok to melt. Stir in the cabbage and cook until just done. Mix together the vinegar and the spices and cook for another couple of minutes. Set aside. Place the remaining butter into the pan. Stir in the meat and cook until brown and cooked through. Reduce the heat to Low and stir the cheese through it. Cook, stirring continuously, until the cheese is completely melted. Put the cream in and let it cook until it thickens a little. Stir the cabbage in and heat everything through. Adjust the seasoning as you like. Serve with the chopped parsley.

15. Indian Stir-Fried Cabbage

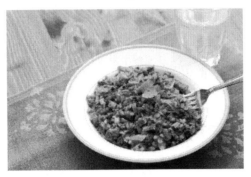

Serves 4

Ingredients

- 1/3 pound farm butter
- 1 2/3 pounds green cabbage
- 1 1/3 pounds ground pork
- 1 teaspoon onion powder
- 1 teaspoon table salt
- ¼ teaspoon powdered black pepper
- 1 tablespoon red curry paste
- 1 tablespoon white wine vinegar
- ½ mild onion, chopped up nice and finely
- 1 cup mayo
- 8 tablespoons fresh cilantro

Method

Coarsely grate the cabbage and set your stove to Med-High. Melt half the farm butter in a wok and stir the cabbage through. Cook until just done. Mix together the vinegar and the spices and fry for another minute or two. Set to the one side. Using the same frying pan, melt the remaining half of the farm butter. Stir in the curry paste, the onion and the garlic and cook for a minute or so. Stir in the meat and cook until it is completely done. Stir the cabbage through and cook until heated all the way through. Serve with the cilantro and the mayo.

16. Burger and Fries with Goat Cheese

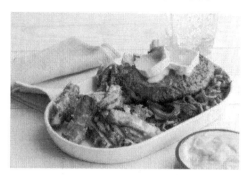

Serves 4

Ingredients Tomato-Flavored Mayo

- Seasoning to taste
- 1 tablespoon tomato paste
- 1 1/3 cups mayo
- 1 pinch cayenne pepper

Ingredients for the Fries

- 1 1/3 cups almond flour
- 1 zucchini
- 1 1/3 cups fresh Parmesan
- 1 teaspoon table salt
- 1 teaspoon onion powder
- ½ teaspoon pepper
- 3 tablespoons olive oil
- 2 eggs

Ingredients for the Burger

- 2 red onions
- 1 ounces of farm butter
- 1 tablespoon red wine vinegar
- Seasoning to taste
- 1 2/3 pounds beef, minced
- 3½ ounces of lettuce
- 3½ ounces of goat cheese

Method

Set your oven at 400. Start by making the tomato-flavored mayo – mix all the ingredients together and put it to one side. Make the fries next. Grease a baking tin and line with baking paper. Beat the eggs and stir in the flour, onion powder, Parmesan and seasoning as required. Chop the zucchini into half lengthwise and deseed it. Chop into fries. Dip the zucchini into the flour and then into the egg. Follow up with a final dip in the flour. Lay the fries out in a single layer on the baking tin. Put in the oven and cook for about 25 minutes or until done. While the fries are in the oven, work on preparing the burgers. Slice up the onions as thinly as possible. Set your stove to Medium and melt your farm butter. You then need to add the onion and cook until soft. Put in the vinegar when the onions are just about done and stir well. Season as you like and put to one side. Season the meat to taste and shape it into patties and fry until done as you like them. Serve on the lettuce with the onions. Put the burgers on top, top with the cheese and mayo and serve.

17. Creamy Spinach and Kale Soup

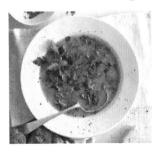

Serves 4

Ingredients

- ½ pound kale
- 3¼ ounces of coconut oil
- ½ pound fresh spinach
- 3⅓ cups coconut milk
- 2 avocados
- Fresh mint as required
- 1 cup of plain water
- 1 teaspoon table salt
- The juice of 1 lime
- ¼ teaspoon powdered black pepper

Method

Set the stove to Med-High and put the coconut oil in a heavy-based pot. Cook the garlic for a minute or so. Stir in the kale and spinach and cook for a few minutes or until just wilted. Take off the heat. Mix in the avocado, the milk, spices and water. Blend until pureed. Mix the lime juice and season to taste.

18. Stir-Fried Turkey

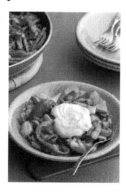

Serves 4

Ingredients for Wasabi mayo

- ½ tablespoon wasabi paste
- ¾ cup mayo
- The zest and juice of 1 lime

Ingredients for the Turkey

- 1 tablespoon fresh ginger, peeled and grated
- 1 pound turkey breast cut into strips
- 1 tablespoon green curry paste
- 1 tablespoon of soy sauce
- ¼ cup coconut oil
- 1 bell pepper of your choice
- 1 pound cabbage
- 3 ounces of celery stalks
- 4 ounces of fresh green beans
- 1 mild onion

Method

Start by making the Wasabi mayo. Mix all the ingredients for the mayo together and put to one side. Mix together the ginger, the curry paste, half of the coconut oil and the soy sauce. Stir the turkey in so that it is completely combined. Put to one side so it can marinate. Chop all of the veggies so that they are bite-sized. Fry the cabbage and cook until it starts to caramelize. Season as you like. Set aside to keep warm. Set your stove to High. Using the same frying pan, fry the meat until it is browned all over. Season as required. Stir in the cabbage and make sure it is heated through. Adjust the seasoning as required. Serve with the mayo.

19. Mexican Casserole Dish

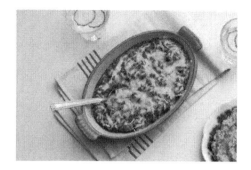

Serves 4

Ingredients

- ½ can crushed tomatoes
- 1½ pounds beef, minced
- 2 ounces of Jalapeños
- 1 cup sour cream
- 7 ounces of Cheddar
- 1 scallion, chopped up nice and finely
- Guacamole to serve
- 2 tablespoons farm butter

Ingredients for the Taco Seasoning

- 2 teaspoons paprika powder
- 2 teaspoons chili powder
- 1 teaspoon powdered cumin
- 1 teaspoon table salt
- 1 pinch cayenne pepper
- 1 – 2 teaspoons onion or garlic powder

Method

Set your oven at 400. Set your stove to Med-High and melt the farm butter in a heavy-based frying pan. Stir in the beef, the tomatoes and the seasoning. Cook until the meat is done. Grease an oven-proof dish and put the beef into it. Mix in the chilis. Sprinkle the cheese over the top. Place on one of the uppermost racks in the oven and cook for about 20 minutes or until the cheese starts to bubble. Chop the scallions up nice and finely and add to the sour cream. Serve with the casserole and guacamole, if being used.

20. Tortillas

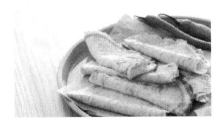

Serves 2

Ingredients

- 2 egg whites
- 2 eggs
- ½ teaspoon table salt
- 6 ounces of cream cheese
- 1 tablespoon coconut flour
- 1 – 2 teaspoons powdered psyllium husks

Method

Set your oven at 400. Mix together the eggs – whites and whole – until fluffy. Mix in the cream cheese. Add the psyllium husks, the flour and the salt. Blend the flour in a little bit at a time until it is all incorporated. Set it aside for a little so that it thickens nicely. Line two baking tins with baking paper and spread the mixture out very thinly so that you have the tortillas. Cook in the oven until they are just done. Watch carefully as they can burn quite easily. When done, add whatever fillings you like.

21. Stroganoff and Low-Carb Rice

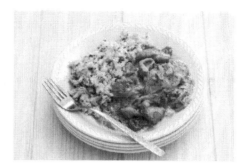

Serves 4

Ingredients

- 2 mild onions
- 1 red bell pepper
- 2 ounces of farm butter
- 1 ounces of sun-dried tomatoes, packed in olive oil
- 1 pound fresh sausages
- 1 tablespoon Dijon mustard
- 2 tablespoons dried thyme
- Seasoning to taste
- 2 tablespoons tomato paste
- 1¼ cups sour cream

Ingredients for the "Rice"

- ¼ cup freshly picked parsley, chopped up nice and finely
- 4 ounces of farm butter
- 1½ pounds cauliflower

Method

Cook the sausages as you normally would and put them one side so that they can cool. Chop the onion and pepper as finely as you can. Set your stove to Medium and melt the farm butter. Stir in the onion and pepper and cook until softened. Chop the sausages up so they are in bite-sized bits and then stir it into the veggies. Fry for a couple of minutes before adding in the remaining ingredients. Bring to the boil and then reduce the heat to Low. Adjust the seasoning as required and serve over the rice.

For the Rice: Coarsely grate the cauliflower. Set the stove to Medium and melt the farm butter. Add the cauliflower and fry it up until is done. Season as required and mix the parsley in just before you serve the food.

22. Chicken Wings and Greens

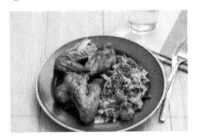

Serves 4

Ingredients for the Chicken Wings

- The zest and juice of ½ an orange
- 3 pounds chicken wings
- ¼ cup olive oil
- ¼ teaspoon cayenne pepper
- 1 teaspoon table salt
- 2 teaspoons ground ginger

Ingredients for the Greens

- 1 cup mayo
- 1½ pounds broccoli
- Seasoning to taste
- ¼ cup chopped fresh dill

Method

Set your oven at 400. Mix together the zest and the juice of the orange in with the spices and the oil. Put it all into a bag that can seal and add the marinade. Shake well so that the wings are completely coated. Set to one side for 10 minutes or so in order to let it marinade. Grease an oven-proof dish and place the chicken in a single layer in the dish. Place the chicken in the middle of the oven and cook for about three quarters of an hour or until cooked through. While the chicken is cooking, prepare the broccoli. Chop up the broccoli and place it in a pot of water. Add salt as required. Cook the broccoli until it is done. Let the broccoli drain thoroughly and set aside for a few minutes to get rid of some of the steam. Serve with the wings and the broccoli.

23. Chicken Casserole

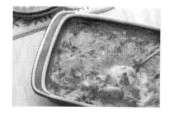

Serves 4

Ingredients

- 2 tablespoons farm butter
- 1 fully roast chicken, cooked
- ½ pound diced bacon
- 2 cups double cream
- ½ pound mushrooms
- 3 – 4 tablespoons ketchup or chili sauce
- 3 tablespoons roasted peanuts (salted)
- Seasoning to taste
- 1 teaspoon yellow curry powder
- 1 banana

Method

Set your oven at 400. Chop up the mushrooms. Set your stove to Medium and melt the farm butter in a heavy-based frying pan. Add the bacon and mushrooms and fry until done. Season as required. Pick the meat off the chicken and slice it up into 1-inch pieces. Grease an oven-proof dish and place the chicken and mushrooms into the frying pan. Peel the banana and slice it up into small bits. Scatter over the chicken mixture and mix well. Whip the cream well until it forms soft peaks. Mix in the curry and the ketchup/ chili sauce. Season as required. Pour it out over the chicken and stir gently. Place in the oven and bake for about 25 minutes or until the dish starts to brown. Serve with the peanuts over the top.

24. Roast Pork and Cauliflower

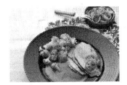

Serves 8

Ingredients for the Pork

- 4 tablespoons natural apple sauce
- 2 pounds pork roast, at room temperature
- 1 tablespoon ground ginger
- ¾ cup of plain
- 1 teaspoon table salt
- 1 tablespoon soy sauce

Ingredients for the Cream sauce

- Seasoning to taste
- 1 cup double cream
- The pan juices leftover from the roast

Ingredients for the Cauliflower

- Seasoning to taste
- 4¼ ounces of farm butter
- 2 pounds of cauliflower, chopped up nice and finely

Method

Set your oven at 350°F. Mix together the spices and the apple and soy sauce. Brush it all over the roast. Grease a roasting tin and place the meat into it. Put it onto one of the lowest racks in the oven. Cook until done. It will be around about 1 ½ hours depending on how big the roast is. The best way to check that it is done is to use a meat thermometer – when the reading at the thickest part of the meat is 165, the meat is done. When the roast is done, place in a foil tent to keep it warm and set to the side and to rest. Take the juices out of the pan and place them in a pot. You want about two cups of the juice. If you don't have enough liquid, add boiling water. Set your stove to Med-High and cook up the juices. Cook until it reduces by around a third. Stir in the cream and bring it to a boil. Reduce the heat to Low and cook for about 10 minutes or until nice and thick. Season as required. Chop up the cauliflower into small bits. Set your stove to Medium and melt the butter. Add in the cauliflower and cook it until it is done. Season as required.

25. Mushroom "Patties" With Fries

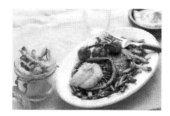

Serves 4

Ingredients

- Seasoning to taste

- 2 ounces of scallions
- 12 cherry tomatoes
- 2 red chili peppers
- 4¼ ounces of farm butter or olive oil
- 4 large Portobello mushrooms

Ingredients for Fries

- 2 cups oil for frying or coconut oil
- salt, to taste
- 1 pound root celery or rutabaga

Ingredients for Chili Aioli

- 1 tablespoon chili powder
- 1 cup mayo
- 2 garlic cloves

Method

Start by making the mayo. Mix all the ingredients for the mayo and set aside so that the flavors can develop. Clean the mushrooms and take out the stems. You can keep the stems to use in another dish. Set your stove to Medium. Add enough farm butter to coat the bottom of a frying pan and cook the mushrooms until done. This takes about 10 minutes per side. Season as required. Remove from the pan and set aside in the warmer drawer. Chop the scallions and the chili up nice and finely. Set your stove to Medium and melt enough butter to cover the base of the pan again. Stir in the scallions and chili and fry for a minute. Add the tomatoes and fry until done. Put into the warmer drawer. Peel the rutabaga/ celery and cut up into fries. Let the fries soak in a bowl of ice-cold water for at least 15 minutes. Pat the fries dry. Heat the oil in a deep saucepan until hot. Cook the fries in batches until they are nice and crisp. Season as required. Drain the excess oil out on paper towels.

26. Chicken Alfredo

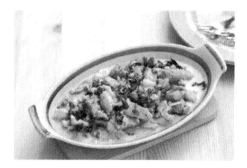

Serves 4

Ingredients

- ⅓ pound bacon, cut into cubes
- 1 ounces of farm butter
- 1⅓ pounds chicken breasts, cut into cubes
- 7 ounces of fresh spinach, chopped up nice and finely
- 4 garlic cloves, crushed
- 3½ ounces of grated Parmesan
- Seasoning to taste
- 1½ pounds cauliflower, chopped up nice and finely
- 2 cups of double cream

Method

Set your stove to Med-High and melt the butter in a frying pan. Add the bacon and fry until it is nice and crisp. Remove the bacon from the pan and put on a plate. In the same pan, fry the garlic and the chicken until the chicken is cooked. Add the spinach and cook until it has just wilted. Remove from the pan and put to one side. Stir in the cream and bring it to a boil, stirring all the while. Stir in the Parmesan, chicken, spinach and the bacon. Season as required. Reduce the heat to Low and cook until it thickens. Boil the cauliflower until done. Season to taste and drain well. Mix with the remaining ingredients and serve.

27. Goulash

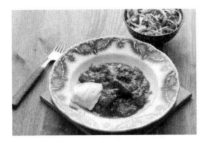

Serves 4

Ingredients for the Goulash

- 2 mild onions
- 4¼ ounces of farm butter
- 2 garlic cloves
- 7½ ounces of root celery
- 2 red bell peppers
- 14 ounces of crushed tomatoes
- 2 pounds chuck roast
- 1 tablespoon tomato paste
- ¾ cup of plain
- 1 tablespoon dried oregano
- 1 teaspoon onion powder
- 1 tablespoon paprika powder
- 1 tablespoon caraway seeds
- ¼ teaspoon powdered black pepper
- 1 teaspoon table salt
- 1 pinch cayenne pepper

Ingredients for Buttery Cabbage

- Seasoning to taste
- 4¼ ounces of farm butter
- 2 pounds green cabbage

For serving

- 1 ounces of freshly picked parsley, chopped up nice and finely
- 1 cup mayo

Method

Chop up the peppers, celery and the peppers finely. Set your stove to Med-High. Melt the butter in a heavy-based frying pan. Add the celery, peppers and onion. Cook until the veggies are done. Stir the garlic into the veggies and cook for another minute or so. Remove the veggies and keep them warm. In a separate pot, mix together the tomatoes, tomato paste, spices and water. Set the stove to Med-High. Cook the tomato mixture until it comes to a boil. Reduce the heat to Low and cook until the mixture thickens. When that is done, chop the meat into 1-inch pieces. If necessary, add more butter so that the pan is coated. Fry the meat until brown. Season as required and then add the vegetables back in. Set the stove to Low and cook the meat for around about two hours, or until done. Check occasionally and add more water if necessary. Season as required. Coarsely grate the cabbage. Set the stove to Med-High and melt the butter in it. Stir in the cabbage and cook until it starts to caramelize. Serve with the goulash and top with some sour cream when serving.

28. Celery Root with Green Beans

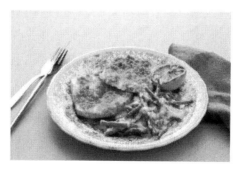

Serves 4

Ingredients

- 2 tablespoons olive oil
- 2 pounds root celery
- ½ teaspoon table salt
- 2 tablespoons coconut flour
- 2 tablespoons desiccated coconut

Ingredients for Creamed Garlic Beans

- 3¼ ounces of farm butter
- 2/3 pound fresh green beans
- 1 cup double cream
- 2 tablespoons chopped freshly picked parsley
- 1 – 2 garlic cloves
- Seasoning to taste
- 2 lemon

Method

Set your oven at 350. Grease a baking sheet and line it with baking paper. Put the root celery onto the sheet and brush with oil. Shake to ensure that the root slices are thoroughly coated. Season as required. Mix the flour and the coconut and sprinkle it over the celery root. Place in the oven and cook for around half an hour or until the celery is cooked through and the breading is nice and brown. While that is cooking, clean and trim the beans. Chop them up into bite-sized pieces. Set the stove to Med-High and melt the farm butter in a saucepan. Crush the garlic and stir into the butter. Add the beans and cook for about 5 minutes. Stir the cream and spices into the butter and bring to the boil. Reduce the heat to Low and allow the cream mixture to thicken nicely. Chop the parsley up nice and finely. And add to the beans just before you serve. Halve the lemon and place in a hot frying pan for a few minutes so that it starts to brown. Squeeze the juice over the top of celery.

29. Mushroom Soup

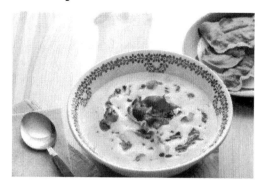

Serves 4

Ingredients

- 1 pound mushrooms
- 1 mild onion
- 4¼ ounces of farm butter
- 5⅓ tablespoons dry white wine
- 1 teaspoon dried thyme
- 7½ ounces of cream cheese
- 1 teaspoon table salt
- 2 cups water
- ¼ teaspoon powdered black pepper
- 1¼ cups double cream
- 4 egg yolks

Ingredients for the Dressing

- Seasoning to taste
- 1 ounces of freshly picked parsley
- 5⅓ tablespoons olive oil

Ingredients for Crisps

- 3¼ ounces of Parma ham

Method

Set your oven at 300. Grease a baking tin and line it with baking paper. Place the ham on the tin in a single layer. Place in the oven on the uppermost rack. Check every few minutes and flip regularly. Cook until the ham crisps. This should take around about a half hour. Chop the onions and mushrooms up. Set your stove to Med-High and add enough butter to cover the base of a heavy-based frying pan. Stir in the mushrooms and onions and cook until they are soft. Season as required and add the thyme. Add in the water, wine and the cheese. Allow the mixture to boil and then reduce the heat to Low. Leave it to simmer for 15 minutes or so, stirring every now and again. While that is cooking, mix together the parsley, oil, and seasoning to taste. Blend with an emulsion blender. Beat the cream until it reaches soft peak stage. Fold the yolks in. Take the soup off the stove and gently fold in the cream mixture. Add the crisps and dressing to taste.

30. Burnt Butter Veggies and Eggs

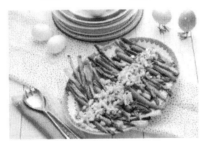

Serves 6

Ingredients

- 1 pound green asparagus
- ¾ pound carrots
- ½ pound scallions
- 2 eggs
- ¼ cup olive oil
- ¼ cup chopped fresh sage
- 3 ounces of farm butter

104

- Seasoning to taste

Method

Set your oven at 450. Clean the veggies well and trim. Grease a baking tin and line with baking paper. Put the veggies into the baking tin in a single layer. Drizzle the olive oil over the veggies and season to taste. Put into the oven and cook for about twenty minutes or until the veggies are cooked through. While the veggies are in the oven, hard boil the eggs. Let them cool off for a bit so that you are able to peel them. Chop up the eggs. Set your stove to Medium and melt the butter in a heavy-based frying pan. Cook until it changes color to a rich brown color and starts to sell a little nutty. Plate the veggies and pour the butter over the top. Finish off with the eggs.

31. Herbed Lamb Chops

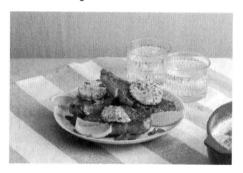

Serves 4

Ingredients

- 1 tablespoon farm butter
- 8 lamb chops
- Herbed farmed butter
- 1 tablespoon olive oil
- Seasoning to taste
- 1 lemon

Method

Set your stove to Medium. Cut the fat on the meat every inch or so to prevent it from curling when cooking. Melt the plain farm butter in a heavy-based frying pan and fry the chops until done – this will normally take about 4 minutes per side. Serve with fresh lemon and the herbed farm butter.

32. Keto Gratin

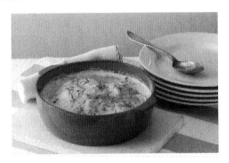

Serves 4

Ingredients

- ½ mild onion
- 1½ pounds turnip
- 1 garlic clove, crushed
- 1¾ ounces of farm butter
- 8 tablespoons freshly picked chives, chopped up nice and finely
- A pinch powdered black pepper
- 1¼ cups double cream
- ½ teaspoon table salt
- 7 ounces of Cheddar, grated

Method

Set your oven at 400. Clean and peel the turnip and the onion. Slice into wafer-thin slices. Snip the chives nice and finely. Grease an oven-proof dish and layer the turnip, the onion, garlic, and cheese. Season each layer as required and be sure to leave some cheese for the top layer. Before putting the last layer of cheese on, pour the cream over the top. Top with the cheese and cook until done. This will take upwards of half an hour.

33. Red Pesto Chops

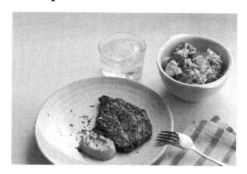

Serves 4

Ingredients

- ⅓ pound mayo
- 2 tablespoons farm butter
- 4 pork chops
- 4 tablespoons red pesto

Method

Set your stove to Medium and spread three tablespoons of the pesto over the chops. Distribute it evenly on both sides. Melt the farm butter in a heavy-based saucepan and fry the chops for about 8 minutes. Reduce the heat to Low and cook for a further 4 minutes. Flip at least once during cooking and cook until done to your liking. While that is cooking, mix together a tablespoon of the pest and the mayo. Serve on the side.

34. Cauliflower Soup with Crumbled Pancetta

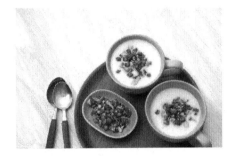

Serves 4

Ingredients

- 1 pound cauliflower
- 3¾ cups chicken stock
- 7¾ ounces of cream cheese
- 4 ounces of farm butter
- 1 tablespoon Dijon mustard
- Seasoning to taste
- 1 tablespoon farm butter
- 7¾ ounces of bacon, diced
- 3½ ounces of pecan nuts
- 1 teaspoon paprika powder

Method

Cut the cauliflower into smaller bits. Keep aside about a handful so that you can garnish the soup later. Set your stove to Med-High. Melt some farm butter in a large saucepan and add the bacon. Cook until crispy. Remove the bacon and melt more farm butter. Remove from the heat. Mix in the cream and mustard and stir well. Next, put the cauliflower in a pot with the stock and cook until done. Add in the cream mixture. Blend until smooth. Serve with the reserved cauliflower and the bacon.

35. Beef Stroganoff

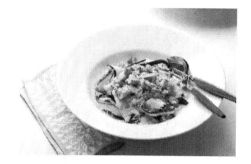

Serves 4

Ingredients

- 3 tablespoons farm butter
- 1 pound beef, minced
- 1 mild onion
- 1 tablespoon dried thyme
- ½ pound mushrooms
- 2 cups sour cream
- ½ teaspoon table salt
- ½ pound blue cheese
- 1 pinch powdered black pepper

Ingredients for the Fettucine

- Seasoning to taste
- Farm butter
- 4 small to medium sized zucchinis

Method

Clean the onion and then chop it up nice and finely. Set your stove to Medium. Melt the farm butter and cook the onion till it starts to soften. Stir in the meat and cook until it is brown. Chop up the mushroom and stir it into the mince. Cook until the mushrooms have softened. Add the seasoning and thyme. Crumble up the blue cheese and stir it into the stroganoff. Stir in the cream and bring the mixture to a boil. Reduce the heat to Low and cook for about 10 minutes, stirring every now and again. Make the fettucine next. Chop the zucchini in half along its length. Remove the seeds and then cut the zucchini into wafer thin slices or spiralize it. Place the zucchini into a pot full of water. Season to taste. Set the stove to Med-High. Put the zucchini on and bring the water to a boil. Drain the zucchini well and then stir in the farm butter. Season as you like and serve straightaway.

36. Wrapped Shrimp Salad

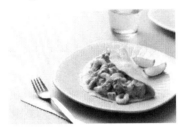

Serves 2

Ingredients for the Wraps

- Seasoning to taste
- 1 ounce of farm butter
- 4 eggs

Ingredients for the Salad

- 1 teaspoon lime juice
- 2 avocados
- 6 ounces of shrimps, cleaned, peeled and cooked
- 1 celery stalk
- ½ apple
- 1 red chili pepper, chopped up nice and finely
- 8 tablespoons fresh cilantro
- 1 cup mayo

Method

Start by making the wraps. Beat the eggs and season them as required. Set your stove to Medium and melt one ounce of the farm butter in a crepe pan. When the butter has just melted, pour in half the egg mixture. Cook until done – they just need to be cooked through, not browned. Do the second wrap in the same way.

For the Salad: Peel the avocado and cube it. Put into the bowl and pour the lime juice over it. Chop the celery and apple nice and finely. Mix in with the avocado. Chop the chili and cilantro up nice and finely. Stir into the salad. Finish off by adding the mayo and shrimps. Season to taste.

37. Pork Chops and Cheese

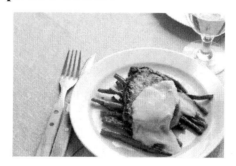

Serves 4

Ingredients

- 2 tablespoons farm butter
- 4 pork chops
- Seasoning to taste
- 1 tablespoon farm butter
- 1¼ cups double cream
- 7 ounces of blue cheese
- 7 ounces of fresh green beans

Method

Set the stove to Medium and melt the cheese in a small saucepan. Add the cream and cook for another few minutes. Cook the chops as you normally do and add seasoning as you require. Set the meat aside and mix the juices from the pan into the sauce. Check to see if you need to adjust the seasoning. Trim the beans. Place in a pot with enough water to cover them. Add salt as required and cook the beans until they are done. Serve the chops on a plate of the beans with the sauce over the top.

38. Pierogis

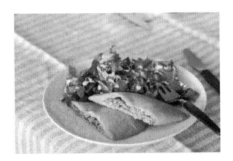

Serves 4

Ingredients for the Filling

- 2 garlic cloves, chopped up nice and finely
- 2 tablespoons farm butter
- 1 shallot, chopped up nice and finely
- 2 ounces of bacon
- 3¼ ounces of mushrooms
- 2 ounces of fresh spinach
- 1/3 pound cream cheese
- ¼ teaspoon pepper
- 2 ounces of Parmesan, grated
- ½ teaspoon table salt

Ingredients for the Pierogi dough

- 4 tablespoons coconut flour
- 8 tablespoons almond flour
- ½ teaspoon table salt
- 1½ cups cheese, grated
- 1 teaspoon baking powder
- 1 egg
- 2 2/3 ounces of farm butter
- 1 beaten egg, for brushing the top of the pierogi

Method

Make the filling first. Set your stove to Med-High. Melt the butter and add the spinach, mushrooms, bacon, garlic and shallots. Season as required. Reduce the heat to Low and stir in the cream and the cream cheese. Cook for a couple of minutes and then set aside. Now make the pierogis. Set your oven at 350. Mix the dry ingredients. Beat the egg and add it to the dry ingredients. Divide up the dough in 4 evenly-sized balls. Flatten the dough balls until they are about 1/5 of an inch thick. Shape into rounds. Divide the filling up between the dough rounds. Fold the pieces in half and press down the open edges with a fork to properly seal the dough. Brush with egg or with milk and put in the oven for around 20 minutes or so. Bake until the pierogis are crisp and looking brown.

39. Salmon Tandoori with Cucumber Sauce

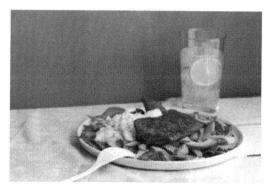

Serves 4

Ingredients

- 2 tablespoons coconut oil
- 1 tablespoon Tandoori spice
- 1½ pounds salmon,

Cucumber Sauce

- ½ cucumber, grated
- 1¼ cups sour cream
- 2 garlic cloves, crushed
- ½ teaspoon table salt
- The juice of ½ lime

Ingredients for the Salad

- 1 mild bell pepper
- 3½ ounces of arugula
- 3 scallions
- The juice of 1 lime
- 2 avocados

Method

Set the oven at 350. Mix up two tablespoons of the oil and stir in the Tandoori spices. Brush it onto the salmon. Grease an oven-proof dish and put the salmon into it. Cook for about 15 minutes or until the salmon is cooked. Squeeze as much juice out of the cucumber as you can. Mix in all the ingredients for the sauce. Make the salad by chopping all the salad ingredients and mixing them. Plate the salad, top it with the sauce and then finish it off with the fish.

40. Steak Béarnaise

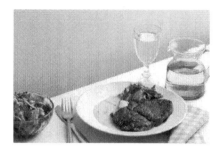

Serves 4

Ingredients

- Seasoning to taste
- 2 tablespoons farm butter
- 4 ribeye steaks

Ingredients for the Béarnaise sauce

- Seasoning to taste
- 2 teaspoons white wine vinegar
- 4 egg yolks
- 2 pinches onion powder
- ⅔ pound farm butter
- 2 tablespoons freshly picked tarragon, chopped up nice and finely

Salad

- 2 ounces of lettuce
- 2 ounces of arugula

Method

Start by making the sauce. Beat the egg yolks until well mixed. In a separate bowl, mix together the onion powder, the tarragon and the vinegar. Set your stove to Medium-High and place the vinegar mixture in a small saucepan. Bring it to the boil and cook for around about 4 minutes or until the sauce has reduced. Scoop out the tarragon. Reduce the heat to Low and add the egg yolks, beating continuously. The sauce is ready when you can see what looks like ribbons forming. Whisk in the butter a little at a time. Don't let the mixture come to the boil again – remove from the stove if this starts to happen. Season to taste and transfer to a bowl to stop it from cooking more and set aside were it can stay warm. Cook the steaks to your liking and serve on a bed of lettuce and arugula. Top off with the sauce.

41. Risotto with Mushrooms

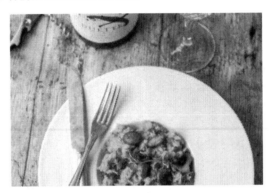

Serves 4

Ingredients

- 1 cup vegetable stock
- 1 cauliflower
- 8¾ ounces of mushrooms
- 1 shallot
- 2 garlic cloves
- 1 cup double cream
- ¾ cup coarsely grated Parmesan
- ¾ cup white wine
- 3½ ounces of farm butter
- Freshly picked thyme, to taste
- Seasoning to taste

Method

Slice the mushrooms into thin slices. Chop the garlic and the onion nice and finely. Set your stove to Med-High and melt the farm butter in a heavy-based frying pan. Stir in the onions and cook until translucent. Add the mushrooms and garlic and fry until soft. Grate up the cauliflower roughly and put it into the pan with the onions and mushrooms. Stir in half of wine and the stock. Bring it to a boil and then reduce the heat to Low. Simmer until the liquid has reduced by half. Add what is left of the wine and stir in the cream. Allow the mixture to simmer until most of the liquid has cooked out.

42. Pork Chops with Green Bean and Avocado on The Side

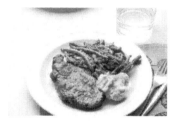

Serves 4

Ingredients for the Pork Chops

- 2 tablespoons olive oil
- 4 pork shoulder chops
- 2 tablespoons mild chipotle paste
- ½ teaspoon table salt

Ingredients for the Garlic Farm Butter

- 1 garlic clove
- 4¼ ounces of farm butter, softened
- ½ teaspoon table salt
- ¼ teaspoon paprika powder

- ¼ teaspoon powdered black pepper

For The Beans And Avocado

- ⅔ pound fresh green beans
- 2 tablespoons olive oil
- ½ teaspoon table salt
- 2 avocados
- Freshly picked cilantro (to taste)
- ¼ teaspoon powdered black pepper
- 6 scallions
- Pepper to taste

Method

Mix together the oil, the salt and the chipotle paste. Brush it all over the meat and leave it to marinade for a minimum of 20 minutes. Set your oven at 400. Grease a roasting tin and place the chops into it. Place in the oven for at least half an hour, or until the chops are cooked. Turn halfway through the cooking time. While that is in the oven, move onto the garlic farm butter. Crush the garlic and blend it with the spices and the butter. Put to one side while you make the beans. Chop up the onion nice and finely. Scoop out the flesh of the avocado and thoroughly mash it. Clean and trim the beans. Set your stove to Med-High and heat up the oil in a heavy-based frying pan. Cook the beans, stirring often, until they start to brown. Reduce the heat and season to taste. Stir the avocado and onion into the bean mixture and cook until heated through. Serve with the cilantro as a garnish.

43. Crunchy Lemon Cabbage Wedges

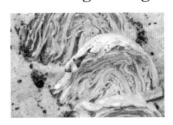

Serves 4

Ingredients

- Seasoning to taste
- 2 tablespoons olive oil
- 1 green cabbage
- 3 tablespoons lemon juice

Method

Set your oven at 440. Grease a baking tin. Divide the cabbage into halves and then halve each of these halves. Mix together the lemon juice and the oil and brush this all over the cabbage. Season to taste. Put in the oven for about 15-20 minutes or until the sides crisp up and look a little charred.

Chapter 4: Snacks

1. Pâté

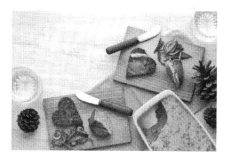

Serves 4

Ingredients

- 1 garlic clove
- 1 red onion
- ½ pound farm butter

- 1 tablespoon tomato paste
- 2 tablespoons brandy or port wine (optional)
- 1 pound chicken livers

Ingredients for the Farm Butter

- 1 teaspoon powdered black pepper
- 1 tablespoon dried thyme
- 4¼ ounces of farm butter

Method

Chop up the garlic and onion nice and finely. Set your stove to Med-High. Place two tablespoonfuls of farm butter into a large frying pan and cook the garlic and onions until they are soft. Take the garlic and onions out of the pan. Set the stove to High and add in some more farm butter. Put the liver in the pan and make sure that it is browned on all sides. Add the liquor and seasoning as required. Reduce the heat and cook until the juices are reduced by half. Mix in the onion mixture and blend until smooth. Mix in with the tomato paste and farm butter. Line a 7" x 8" with baking paper. Spread the pate out over the baking sheet in an even layer. Make the topping next. Set the stove to Medium. Place the farm butter in little saucepan and let the butter melt. Scoop off the clarified butter that will rise to the surface. Discard the remaining butter. Add the pepper and thyme. Pour over the top of the pâté and put into the refrigerator to set.

2. Garlic Bread

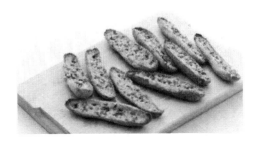

Serves 4

Ingredients for the Bread

- 5 tablespoons powdered psyllium husks
- 1¼ cups almond flour
- 2 teaspoons baking powder
- 3 egg whites
- 2 teaspoons apple cider vinegar
- 1 teaspoon table salt
- 1¼ cups boiling water

Garlic Farm Butter

- 1 garlic clove, minced
- 4 ounces of farm butter, at room temperature
- ½ teaspoon table salt
- 2 tablespoons freshly picked parsley, chopped up nice and finely

Method

Set your oven at 350. Mix together all the dry ingredients. Set your stove to Med-High and put the water in a pot. Bring the water to a boil and mix in the egg whites and the vinegar, whisking all the time. Mix with the dry ingredients until you get a smooth dough. Divide the dough into 10 evenly-sized pieces and shape them so that they look like hot dog buns. Grease a baking tray and set the buns out on it. Leave space all round so that there is space for them to double. Put it in the oven on one of the lower racks for about three quarters of an hour or until they sound hollow when you tap on them. In the meantime, mix up the garlic farm butter. Mix together all of the ingredients well and store in the refrigerator. Remove the buns and allow it to cool. Remove the butter and serve on the buns when the buns are cool. Set your oven to 425. Place the garlic bread slices in the oven until they crisp up and are golden.

3. Ranch Dip

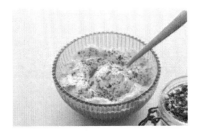

Serves 4

Ingredients

- 8 tablespoons sour cream
- 1 cup mayo
- ¼ teaspoon powdered black pepper
- 1 teaspoon dried chives or dried tarragon
- 1 teaspoon dried dill
- 1 teaspoon dried parsley
- ½ teaspoon garlic powder
- ½ teaspoon table salt
- ½ teaspoon onion powder

Method

It is best to make this the night before you want to use it so that the flavors can develop properly. If that is not an option, give it at least 2 hours. Mix together all of the ingredients and then store in the refrigerator.

4. Zucchini Crisps

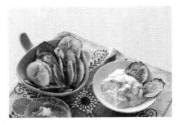

Serves 4

Ingredients

- Table salt to taste
- 2 tablespoons olive oil
- 2 zucchinis

Method

Set your oven at 250. Grate the zucchini coarsely. Lay the slices on a large baking sheet and salt them. Set aside for 15 minutes and then dab off any extra moisture. Grease a couple of clean baking sheets and line them with baking paper. Set the zucchini out on the baking paper. Brush the zucchini with olive oil. Put them in the oven for an hour or until crispy. Do watch carefully to ensure that the zucchini does not burn. Let them cook off and then serve.

5. Blue-Cheese Dressing

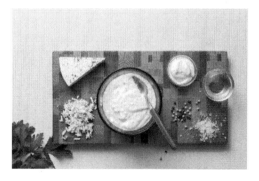

Serves 4

Ingredients

- Double cream (optional)
- ¾ cup Greek yogurt
- 4¾ ounces of blue cheese
- 8 tablespoons mayo

- Seasoning to taste
- 2 tablespoons freshly picked parsley, chopped up nice and finely

Method

Crumble up the cheese and mix everything together. Season as required and allow to sit for an hour to let the flavors develop.

6. Guacamole

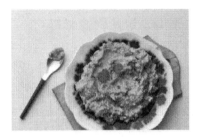

Serves 4

Ingredients

- Seasoning to taste
- 1 – 2 garlic cloves, crushed
- 2 ripe avocados
- ½ lime, the juice
- ½ white onion
- 3 tablespoons olive oil
- 1 tomato, diced
- 5 1/3 tablespoons fresh cilantro

Method

Remove the flesh from the avocados and mash. Stir in the lime juice. Grate the onion nice and finely and stir into the avocado mixture. Mix in the olive oil, cilantro and tomato. Season as required and serve.

7. Salami Chips

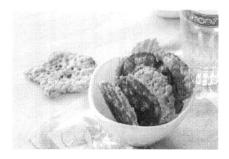

Serves 4

Ingredients

- 1 teaspoon paprika powder
- 4½ ounces of grated Parmesan
- 3¼ ounces of salami, about 20 slices

Method

Set your oven at 450. Grease a baking tray and line it with baking paper. Put the salami onto the baking sheet. Top each slice with some cheese and season as required. Put into the oven and bake until the cheese starts to crisp up. Allow to cool before serving.

8. Cheese Crisps

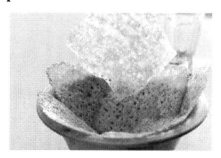

Serves 4

Ingredients

- ½ teaspoon paprika powder
- ½ pound Cheddar, sliced

Method

Set your oven at 400. Grease a baking sheet and line it with baking paper. Put the Cheddar onto the sheet. Season with the paprika and bake for around 8 minutes or until the cheese is crispy. Allow the crisps to cool before serving.

9. Onion Rings

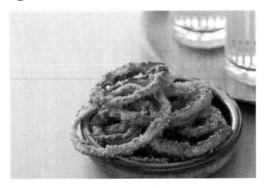

Serves 4

Ingredients

- 1 egg
- 1 big onion
- 1 cup almond flour
- 1 teaspoon garlic powder
- 8 tablespoons fresh Parmesan, grated
- ½ tablespoon chili powder
- 1 tablespoon olive oil
- 1 pinch salt

Method

Set your oven at 400. Slice the onion up into 1/5 inch rings. Mix all of the dry ingredients to. Mix an egg in a well. Dip your onions into the batter and then into the flour. Line a large baking tin with baking paper and lay out the onion rings. Bake for about 15 minutes in the oven or until they are crisp.

Conclusion

I hope that you have enjoyed these recipes and that you will have been inspired to try them out for yourself.

Once you understand something about how ketogenic recipes work, you can start to mix and match and experiment on your own.

With the great recipes in this book, you probably won't even feel like you are on diet. Losing weight could not be any easier.

Best of luck!

Final Words

I would like to thank you for downloading my book and I hope I have been able to help you and educate you on something new.

If you have enjoyed this book and would like to share your positive thoughts, could you please take 30 seconds of your time to go back and give me a review on my Amazon book page!

I greatly appreciate seeing these reviews because it helps me share my hard work!

Again, thank you and I wish you all the best!

Last Chance to Get YOUR Bonus!

FOR A LIMITED TIME ONLY – Get Sarah's best-selling book *"The #1 Weight Loss Guide: The ONLY Book You Will Need to Read to Lose Weight FOREVER!"* absolutely FREE!

Readers who have read this bonus book as well have seen the greatest changes in their health and weight loss both *QUICKLY & EASILY* and have improved overall fitness levels – so it is *highly recommended* to get this bonus book.

Once again, as a big thank-you for downloading this book, I'd like to offer it to you *100% FREE for a LIMITED TIME ONLY!*

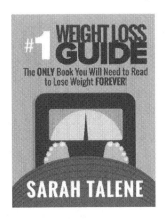

To download your FREE copy, go to:

TopFitnessAdvice.com/Freebie

Disclaimer

This book and related sites provide wellness management information in an informative and educational manner only, with information that is general in nature and that is not specific to you, the reader. The contents of this site are intended to assist you and other readers in your personal wellness efforts. Consult your physician regarding the applicability of any information provided in our sites to you.

Nothing in this book should be construed as personal advices or diagnosis, and must not be used in this manner. The information provided about conditions is general in nature. This information does not cover all possible uses, actions, precautions, side-effects, or interactions of medicines, or medical procedures. The information in this site should not be considered as complete and does not cover all diseases, ailments, physical conditions, or their treatment.

You should **consult with your physician before beginning any exercise, weight loss, or healthcare program**. This book **should not** be used in place of a call or visit to a competent health-care professional. You should consult a health care professional before adopting any of the suggestions in this book or before drawing inferences from it.

Any decision regarding treatment and medication for your condition should be made with the advice and consultation of a qualified health care professional. If you have, or suspect you have, a health-care problem, then you should immediately contact a qualified health care professional for treatment.

No Warranties: The authors and publishers don't guarantee or warrant the quality, accuracy, completeness, timeliness, appropriateness or suitability of the information in this book, or of any product or services referenced by this site.

The information in this site is provided on an "as is" basis and the authors and publishers make no representations or warranties of any kind with respect to this information. This site may contain inaccuracies, typographical errors, or other errors.

Liability Disclaimer: The publishers, authors, and other parties involved in the creation, production, provision of information, or delivery of this site specifically disclaim any responsibility, and shall not be held liable for any damages, claims, injuries, losses, liabilities, costs, or obligations including any direct, indirect, special, incidental, or consequences damages (collectively known as "Damages") whatsoever and howsoever caused, arising out of, or in connection with the use or misuse of the site and the information contained within it, whether such Damages arise in contract, tort, negligence, equity, statute law, or by way of other legal theory.